Yoga and the Hindu Tradition

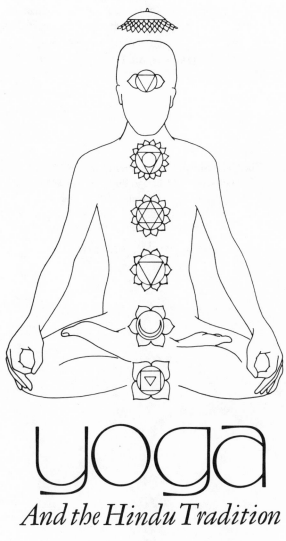

yoga

And the Hindu Tradition

Jean Varenne

Translated from the French by Derek Coltman

The University of Chicago Press

Chicago and London

Jean Varenne is professor of Sanskrit and Indian civilization
at the University of Provence. The present work first appeared under
the title *Le yoga et la tradition hindoue,*

. . . . oisirs

s, Chicago 60637
The University of Chicago Press, Ltd., London
© 1976 by The University of Chicago

7877767574   987654321

Library of Congress Cataloging in Publication Data

Varenne, Jean.
  Yoga and the Hindu tradition.

  Translation of Le yoga et la tradition hindoue.
  "Yoga Darshana Upanishad": p.
  Bibliography: p.
  Includes index.
  1. Yoga.   I. Upanishads.   Darsanopanisad.   English.
Selections.   II. Title.
B132.Y6V2913   181'.45   75-19506
ISBN 0-226-85114-1

Contents

Illustrations

Preface

Yoga—a with-it word perpetually catching the eye from posters, from the covers of garishly printed magazines, and, needless to say, from publishers' catalogs. It is also a good conversational standby: "I do yoga every Friday afternoon, I find it relaxes me"; someone else "does yoga" to help his bad back; another "to keep a clear head at work." Almost everywhere you can find flourishing "schools of yoga" that teach a sort of Swedish drill interspersed with pauses for breathing: "Breathe in as deeply as you can, hold it, relax." The teacher twists himself into bizarre contorsions, pulls his legs behind his neck, ties his fingers into strange knots. Awed and amazed, the clients themselves venture no further than simply sitting cross-legged on the floor; and even that they find uncomfortable and difficult to keep for very long.

In other circles, things are different: we find nothing but scorn for what the businessmen and middle-class housewives doing gymnastics for their sciatica call their "yoga." These others know that yoga is an initiatory wisdom that has come to us from the very depths of time (and space—India is not all that close, even by jet) and is, in consequence, occult, reserved for secret societies. In these circles one is no longer a paying client but a "disciple"; one practices a ritual, becomes a vegetarian, meditates on the Absolute. "Master, when I am meditating I see huge orange flames; is that good?" The master makes some learned reply, suitable to his elevated position, and then delivers a sermon, whereupon the disciples thank him and return to their occupations—office work, studies, housekeeping. These are the people who publish esoteric magazines and write articles in which they drop names like Ramakrishna, Aurobindo, and so on. The dream of these disciples is to travel to India and become part of an ashram, as the Beatles once did.

For some, the dream becomes a reality; they go and spend their summer vacation at Rishikesh, where the Ganges transmutes itself from mountain torrent into majestic river. And what do they find? A circus! Dozens (hundreds?) of gurus, all comfortably ensconced and vying with one another for clients, each only too ready to explain why his rivals are worthless ignoramuses. If the visitor has been sent out under the aegis of a reputable organization, however, things are different; the address he was handed in Europe turns out to be that of a vast monastery, an institution run on the most modern lines, often air-conditioned cells. The food in the refectory—sorry, the cafeteria!—is vegetarian, but the hard cash price of bed and board is decidedly high. During the day, disciples work under the guidance of assistants; then in the evening everyone congregates around the guru. Sitting on a dais, bedecked with garlands of flowers, the master receives his tributes of fruit and incense; he is worshiped like a god with cries of *Jay gurudev!* ("Long live our holy master!") as the assembly prostrates itself before him. Some, the most fervent of his votaries, are permitted the honor of touching his feet.

His actual teaching is rather like the kind of sermon that might be given in a church in a large resort town; the disciples are so numerous and from such a vast variety of backgrounds that it is impossible for the guru ever to venture beyond the most elementary philosophical propositions spiced with a great deal of moralistic advice ("It is time to pull ourselves together, to give God his rights, to make the necessary personal effort!" etc.). Was it worth the personal effort of traveling all the way to India just to hear that? During the day, it is true, the guru does receive some disciples individually, offering moral guidance with an admixture of practical advice on "how to achieve liberation." Nevertheless, it is the atmosphere that really counts; the disciple is surrounded by other devotees, by the heady scent of jasmine, by an amazing calm. He quickly becomes accustomed to remaining silent in the presence of the master while the latter meditates in the midst of his closest disciples, and when he returns to Europe he is still a little dazed by it all.

But yoga itself? Even the most naive are well aware that they have come nowhere near it, and the better-informed know only too well that the weeks they have spent at Rishikesh (or Pondicherry, or one of a hundred other places) are not even the beginning of a novitiate. For yoga is something that can be undertaken only after a long probationary period, a novitiate culminating in a specific ceremony during which the accepted aspirant solemnly renounces the world (in the most concrete way, too—by donating his entire worldly possessions to the community into which he is received; hence the incredible wealth of the best-known ashrams). Many of these would-be disciples end up feeling duped and disappointed: "Why weren't we warned? We could have avoided wasting our time." Some never quite shake off their nostalgia for a spiritual adventure incompatible with the realities of their daily lives, and sometimes suffer from obvious symptoms of frustration as a consequence.

I trust that this book will help to spare others a similar disenchantment. Those who read it will come to realize that it is in fact dishonest to reduce yoga to some sort of physical training, or merely to an occult doctrine; it is a "world view," a *Weltanschauung* that comprehends reality in its totality—material as well as spiritual—and provides the foundation for certain practices intended to enable those worthy of it to integrate themselves totally into that reality, if not to transcend it. It is true that there is an element of the occult involved in this doctrine, because it requires a great deal of assimilating and because the help of a spiritual guide is indispensable if one is to succeed in doing so concretely. But there is nothing actually secret about it, the texts have all been published and the ashrams are open to anyone who presents himself. As for the gymnastic part of it, that is just one prescribed practice among many; the most picturesque, admittedly, but not the most important.

My aim, then, is to "rehabilitate" yoga, as it were. And my method will be simply to present the theory of classical yoga, in its entirety, by following the great classical texts on the subject step by step, and by quoting from them freely. The reader will thus be in a position to measure the gulf between the richness of the traditional doctrine and the poverty of so many vapid extrapolations from it. Then he can choose.

This book first appeared in France in November 1973. The present translation differs little from the original, though I have corrected a number of errors in the French edition and taken account of some readers' comments. The bibliography has been entirely recast to meet the needs of English-speaking users. It is not intended to be exhaustive but is limited, instead, to useful works that are easily accessible in bookstores or libraries.

All passages from yoga texts included here were newly translated for the French edition directly from the Sanskrit. They do not of course exempt the reader from referring to existing translations listed in the notes and bibliography. In this respect, English-speaking readers have an advantage, since all the great texts have been available in English for many years. Some of these translations, however, can be improved, and this I have attempted to do, notably with the *Yoga Darshana Upanishad,* appended to this study as an example of the sacred texts to which the traditional masters turn.

Terminology

A great number of Sanskrit words will be encountered during the course of this book. This is the result not of pedantry but of necessity: the categories of thought and underlying culture involved are so different from our own that translations can never be more than very approximate. All these words will be explained in the text or notes and also, where they are used with some frequency, in the glossary.

Pronunciation of Sanskrit words

1. *o* and *e* are always long.
2. *u* is always *oo.*
3. *g* is always hard.
4. *s* is always unvoiced, never *z.*
5. All aspirates are strongly sounded. *H* inside a word (as in *brahman*) is a guttural like the *ch* in Scottish *loch* or the *j* in Spanish *navaja.*

It should be noted that, in accordance with common usage, the forms *yogi, brahmin,* and *avatar* have been used rather than *yogin, brahmana, avatara.* Diacritics have been omitted, both for reasons of economy and because this book has been written largely for nonspecialists. Sanskrit scholars accustomed to more formal transliteration are asked to extend their indulgence.

Introduction

Cut off to the north by the enormous mountain complex of the Himalayas, bounded to the south by an ocean that extends uninterrupted to Antarctica, contained to the east by the interweaving mountain chains of High Burma, India is open only to the west, to Iran, with which it communicates via the bleak passes of the Hindu Kush and the vast, desertlike stretches of Baluchistan. In other words, it is more or less an island or, as the geographers put it, a subcontinent. This insularity has made possible the originality of a culture that has remained profoundly faithful to itself since the dawn of history; and in the case of India that means for some five thousand years. An amazing continuity, almost unique in the world, since apart from India it would seem that China alone can provide evidence of any analogous cultural development, one without breaks and without rejections.

The only remaining testimony to the prestigious civilization of ancient Egypt lies buried in archaeological remains; which meant that the inhabitants of the Nile valley, converted to Islam thirteen centuries ago, had to wait for Champollion to decipher the hieroglyphics before they could know anything of the beliefs of their distant ancestors. Yet during all that time Hindu families continued, and still continue today, to venerate the selfsame Vishnu who was celebrated in the archaic hymns of the *Rig Veda* as long ago as the second millennium B.C.![1] And even ten centuries earlier than that, about 3,000 B.C., the builders of the Indus valley cities were stamping their earthenware seals—found in such abundance in the excavations at Mohenjo-Daro and Harappa—with the figures of gods that are already Hindu, as can clearly be seen from the famous "proto-Shiva,"[2] seated in the typical cross-legged position and surrounded by Shiva's customary escort of wild animals.

It would be impossible to overemphasize this exceptional durability of a civilization that is extremely difficult to conceive of as mortal. And certainly the Hindus themselves would be the last to subscribe to the notion that all cultures have a limited life-span. That is the product of

Western minds trained at an early age to write essays on "The Causes of the Fall of the Roman Empire," of a Christian or a Moslem faith proud of the fact that its first believers once repudiated pagan polytheism, and therefore prone to assume that all civilizations are perishable the same way as human beings themselves. To the tradition-minded Hindu, on the other hand, such revolutions are inconceivable; for him, the religion he professes has no beginning and no end; it had no founder, and it lies in no one's power to attack or breach it. It is the eternal norm (in Sanskrit, *sanatana dharma*), the universal law, the supreme religion. Being absolute, it cannot be modified in any way and remains identical to itself down the ages.

This does not mean, of course, that the Hindus are incapable of objectivity or that they are unaware of the fact that dharma has in the past been subjected to defeats—even within India itself—by Islam, for example, and even before that by Buddhism. But such things are merely "signs of the times" among so many others, warning us that we have now entered the iron age, whose ineluctable outcome must be the end of this universe. However, our world will vanish only in order that it may be reborn, in accordance with the law of cosmic cycles, and the eternal dharma will remain the same in the world to come, just as it was the same in the world that preceded ours. And since each successive universe develops like a living organism, its vitality ebbing as time passes, the decline of each universe can be measured by the degree to which the individuals in it have moved away from the eternal norm at any given moment. Thus all living beings will observe dharma in the golden age,[3] three-quarters of them in the silver age, only half in the bronze age, and barely a quarter at the onset of the iron age. Seen from this point of view, the fact that men could choose to reject dharma, even on the supremely holy soil of India itself, and give their allegiance to Islam or to our own Western values, must surely be a sign that the end of time is near. And when the last brahmin has poured his ritual oblation into the sacred fire for the last time, then the sun will rise no more.

We are a long way from our customary categories of thought, deep in an exotic cultural land. But any bewilderment this "culture shock" may cause can only be salutary here. Yoga, as we shall see, is a discipline that constitutes one of the essential dimensions of traditional Hinduism, and to attempt to learn anything at all about that discipline without first steeping ourselves in the very substance of dharma itself would be to condemn ourselves to understanding nothing about it at all. Which is why my first long section is devoted to a straightforward exposition of the main lines of force that dictate the structure of the Hindu tradition. Not that I aim to say everything there is to be said about that tradition. No one book could possibly do that, and it would in any case mean going beyond the bounds of our subject, since yoga, though it does indeed lie at the very heart of Hindu culture, by no means represents that heart entirely. I shall therefore content myself with providing a broad background, then highlighting those particular sections of it that will best contribute to the unfolding of our story.

Moreover, what I have just said about the perennial nature of Hinduism also explains my decision to make my presentation of yoga synchronistic—to treat it as though it were truly immutable, both in form and content, and to omit all reference to its history. The Hindus themselves, of course, have no doubt at all about this immutability, since in their eyes yoga is one of the aspects of dharma. But the Western reader, I believe, has the right to ask: Is it conceivable that any discipline as complex as this could really have remained so totally faithful to itself that it is impossible to distinguish between present-day practice and the very earliest teachings? The answer to that question will, I hope, become apparent of its own accord in the course of the exposition that follows. I shall, in addition, offer a kind of historical appraisal in my conclusion; though the very fact that such an appraisal appears as an appendix is sufficient indication that the changes (if changes there have been) have no great significance. Besides, any history of yoga that may possibly exist can clearly not be understood until we know what it is we are talking about. The important thing, therefore, and what this book is essentially trying to do, is to define what yoga itself, the "eternal" yoga, actually is, before looking to see whether the evidence at our disposal either does or does not reveal historical development of any kind.

It is at this point, of course, that we must face the question of whether the discipline we are investigating can actually be described. And, if it can, what method should be used? In deciding, we must keep in mind the fact that yoga is profoundly Indian, and the nature of the documentary evidence available will necessarily reflect that fact. India is a country where the oral tradition holds undisputed sway. Although writing has been known there as long as it has in Iran, for example, the brahmins—the caste responsible for education—have always claimed (and still do claim) that the living word must be the preferred vehicle for the transmission of knowledge. Not merely for technical pedagogic reasons, they add, but above all because Hindu ritual is based upon a belief that the formulas uttered possess an intrinsic magical efficacy of their own. It follows that the Sanskrit manuscripts we possess are never very ancient, which would render the acquisition of any knowledge of ancient India highly problematical had this lacuna not been remedied by the extraordinary fidelity of the aforesaid oral tradition.[4]

Young brahmins, even today, still learn the normative texts of each discipline by heart. Literally thousands of pages are memorized in childhood and adolescence, at an age when for the most part the pupil does not understand the material he is thus passively assimilating. For this very reason the strictest phonetic accuracy must be observed, since a single error of pronunciation could entail unforeseeable consequences. A scrupulous count is kept, not just of the number of words in a given text, but even of the number of syllables, and countless totally artificial divisions and subdivisions are devised (groups of a hundred syllables, for instance) solely to ensure that the reciter is never in danger of forgetting a word or adding one. Pupils are also taught to perform almost acrobatic feats of memory: reciting the text backwards, omitting all the even (or odd) syllables, etc. These feats are in fact nothing more than mnemotechnical exercises and have no value other than their usefulness in that respect; but they do at least provide a guarantee that the doctrinal texts are genuinely nonvariant.

Western experts in the field have long remarked on the fact that the *Veda,* the *Bhagavad-Gita,* and the *Yoga-Sutras* are all entirely lacking in variants, and that their contents could always be easily and infallibly checked by referring to the *pandits*[5] who had learned them by heart in childhood from the mouths of their fathers or a specialized master. This is why, when we speak of "written" evidence with reference to India, we must always remember that we may be referring to texts dating back three or more thousand years (as in the case of certain sections of the *Veda*) of which the oldest known manuscripts may nevertheless only date from, say, the twelfth century after Christ. Let me repeat, however, that the paradox is on the surface only: to Hindus, every aspect of dharma is by definition just as eternal as dharma itself, and its transmission from generation to generation is automatically guaranteed by the chain of initiation and oral education. So that it was not until Islam gained a hold in India, thus creating the risk of a break in that chain, that the guardians of Hindu tradition resigned themselves to fixing it in written form, and even then very incompletely.

It is therefore possible in our day to embark on a study of yoga based on a reading of the discipline's basic texts. In the nineteenth century, the brahmins recognized the possible usefulness of the printing presses the British were importing, and many ashrams equipped themselves with such presses as an aid in diffusing the traditional teachings of which they were the depositories. The use of print made it much easier to spread the basic doctrines of all the dharma-based disciplines, beginning with yoga, among those fitted to receive them (which meant in practice all those—and they were few numerically—who were able to read Sanskrit). It should be added, however, that access to these texts is not quite as easy as might be imagined, even when one is fully conversant with the language in which they are written. One must understand first of all that Indian education—exclusively based on oral transmission, as we have seen—is organized in accordance with a very rigid pedagogical system very much like that used in our own medieval universities, in the time of Saint Thomas Aquinas, for example. In those days theology was taught in the form of sets of linked aphorisms (hence the term *catenae,* "chains," used to denote these rudiments). At the beginning of each lesson the master would give out the "text" for the day, a simple sentence in "telegraphic" style, sometimes even condensed into no more than one word, and then deliver a long commentary on it. Subsequently, the extent of the knowledge the pupils had acquired (and of their latent capacity for becoming masters in their turn) was tested by organized "disputes" or formal debates, veritable intellectual tournaments in which the dialectical gifts of the contestants were displayed and strengthened by use. Their dialectical gifts only, however, since there was absolutely no question of disputing the initial propositions, only of linking, contrasting, or rearranging the positions originally propounded in the masters' commentaries.

This method is the one still employed in Hindu ashrams, which have in fact never known any other. The guru communicates the traditional knowledge in his possession to his duly initiated disciples (after their novitiate) in an exactly identical way: the theme of each lesson is contained in an extremely concise aphorism (two words, three words, often only one) which constitutes, in a sense, its title. The guru then provides a long commentary on it derived from his own acquired knowledge—in other words, mainly from the teachings handed on to him by his own guru.

This is what is called in India the *guru-shishya-parampara,* the "initiatory chain of transmission of traditional knowledge from master to disciple," it being always understood that no other means of communicating that knowledge can exist, since it derives from dharma, the eternal norm. However, it is only the basic aphorism in this case that is held to be "revealed truth"; it alone is intangible and a source of salvation (since to know it, to comprehend it, to assimilate it is to achieve one's salvation). The master's commentary, in contrast, is no more than a means of administering the truth, a method of assisting the disciple. If need be, it is possible to contest it (provided no lack of fidelity to dharma is thereby involved), in particular by setting one interpretation against another, the lessons of one school (meaning one initiatory line) against those of another, etc. This requires knowledge allied to intellectual passion, and only the most advanced disciples, those within sight of becoming gurus in their turn, are capable of holding their own in such tournaments.

In order to convey a concrete notion of what these literally "academic" discussions involve (since the Hindu ashram is not very different from the Platonic academia), let us take as an example the second link in the chain of the *Yoga-Sutras;*[6] it consists of two words only: *yogash chitta-vritti-nirodhah,* which may be translated: "Yoga is the cessation of agitation of the consciousness."

Clearly a statement as elliptical as that is capable of providing ample food for controversy. Is this cessation definitive or temporary (does it involve a true "dissolution of consciousness" as certain schools claim, or simply a temporary suspension of mental activity). Is the agitation that should be made to cease the result of a malfunctioning of one conscious activity (which in that case would merely need correction), or is it an essential property of that consciousness (in which case, is it necessary actually to "destroy" that consciousness)? Is the consciousness to which the revealed text refers identical with thought, or is it a broader category that includes thought (in which case, what ought to "cease": mental activity alone, or all conscious life)?—unless of course this "consciousness" is, on the contrary just one form of thought within the category Thought, and so on. The reader could go on to add innumerable such questions of his own. But he will never succeed single-handed in formulating as many as the various schools of yoga themselves have devised during the past two thousand years and more. However, this one example does make clear both the vast extent and also the strict limits of the commentators' power: none of them is at liberty to doubt that yoga is indeed the cessation of agitation of the consciousness (since that statement derives from revealed truth), but they are all allowed total latitude in interpreting the terms of the statement in their own way.

The final section of this book will make it clear that the interpretations have been both numerous and divergent over the centuries; but it will also show that the resulting arguments are permanent and have hardly developed in all that time. The problems were presented at the outset and the solutions were discovered at once, so that the history of yoga is one of successive "modes" rather than of an evolutive progress, which would be an unthinkable notion within the Hindu cultural context, since the essential truth was given from the start in a totally immutable form. Moreover, the texts of several commentaries that were epoch-making in their day have fortunately come down to us. This happened because the prestige of certain gurus was so great that their teachings were collected by devoted disciples, learned by heart, and then handed on orally until they were eventually written down and later printed. For example, the Ananda Ashrama (which might be translated as "Monastery of the Beatitude"—a pious institution near Poona) produced three commentaries on the basic (and, I must repeat, the only "revealed") text of the *Yoga-Sutras:* those of Vyasa, of Vachaspati Mishra, and of King Bhoja, all three more or less interdependent and all three originally grafted, as it were, onto the stock formed by the sovereign aphorisms attributed to the mythical sage Patanjali—himself merely the human interpreter of divine wisdom.

Other ashrams have likewise bequeathed to us their records of rather more technical teachings centered on the physical exercises that constitute the most familiar aspect of yoga. There is, for instance, the *Hatha-Yoga-Pradipika* and the manuals that derive from it, such as the *Gheranda-Samhita,* the *Shiva-Samhita,* and many others of lesser importance.

So far, we have been considering only those texts that deal with yoga alone, to the exclusion of all the other aspects of dharma. And that is a relatively exceptional position, because Hinduism instinctively prefers encyclopedic works in which the tradition is displayed in all its complexity. Thus we find a richer, more complete, and also more readable presentation of yoga in the great *Puranas* (vast didactic poems in which everything the Hindu should know about dharma is expressed), in the *Bhagavad-Gita* (itself only one constituent part of the great epic poem that tells in a hundred thousand quatrains the story of the war fought among the founding princes of the Indian nation), in the *Tantras* (similar to the *Puranas* but of different inspiration), and lastly in the *Upanishads*.[7]

The *Upanishads* are particularly interesting, since the Hindus themselves look upon them as being what one might call the "Sapiential Books" of the *Veda,* that bible of Hinduism. And that being so, we ought to consider them even more sacred than the *Yoga-Sutras* themselves, a view certainly in keeping with the teaching of traditionalist brahmins. Yoga as such, however, does not occupy the foreground in any but a minority of them, even though it is presented in a diffused or secondary way in almost all. Later on I shall have occasion to point out that this situation is in fact a paradoxical one, since Vedic ideology is actually opposed to yoga as such on many points (and by no means minor ones); but where Western science tends to perceive evidence of evolution, the Hindu tradition prefers to see simply a certain diversity in the relations of its various teachings to dharma, which, needless to say, remains whole and faithful to itself in a realm beyond this superficial conflict produced by varying viewpoints.

Whatever the truth of this problem, however, the evidence of the *Yoga Upanishads* relating to the theory and the practice of classical yoga remains irreplaceable, not merely quantitatively but also on account of the mystic exaltation they succeed in conveying (a feature shared by the *Upanishads* generally, and one that has made them, along with the *Bhagavad-Gita,* probably the best known of all the Hindu scriptures). Here again, some of the commentaries have been preserved, and contemporary masters continue to publish new ones, a proof of the interest they still command.

Thanks to the abundance of the available documentary evidence, it is therefore clear that a study of yoga based solely on a reading of the texts could be both undertaken and justified if that were the only path open to us. But that is equally clearly not the case, since yoga is still very much alive and is still practiced, even in the India of today, in strict accordance with the rules laid down by the traditional texts. It is therefore vital to supplement an attentive analysis of those texts with what we might term "fieldwork." Some readers may even think that the latter method should be the only valid one, since yoga's importance in their view lies in its practice rather than in its theory.

But things are not as simple as that. Of course one could formulate exact descriptions of the physical activities of yogis (adepts or practitioners of yoga)—the taking up of such and such a position, deceleration of the breath rate, squinting at the tip of the nose, and so on—but that would not take us very far unless we simultaneously did our best to understand the purpose of those physical activities. And the answers the masters themselves give invariably involve references back to the discipline's basic texts: "I teach these positions because I belong to such and such an initiatory tradition." No guru, in fact, could ever conceive so preposterous a notion as that of inventing a new position, any more than he could that of altering the details of their execution, no matter how slightly. And this fact greatly restricts the possible interest of field research: the most one can do is to evaluate the fidelity displayed to the tradition, or the ease of execution. And that is still merely scratching the surface; the roots are much deeper down.

The same obstacle recurs if one attempts to elucidate the yogi's motives. "Why do you subject yourself to these exercises?" "Because revelation teaches us that their practice leads to salvation." The adept who has completed the full cycle of traditional practices is convinced that he has achieved his salvation. And how is our observer to reach any decision about that? It is a matter of faith. The pious Hindu venerates the gurus because he believes they have attained salvation. The non-Hindu or the atheist Indian will mock their fatuity or remain skeptical. But the fact itself, whatever the real truth of the matter, cannot be made the object of scientific evaluation. That leaves the direct effects of the exercises—including meditation—on the practitioner's body and mind. At first sight it might appear that there is a possibility here for scientific measurement, for a quantification leading to some kind of objective assessment of yoga. But the electrocardiograms and eletroencephalograms taken by Western scientists have never revealed any meaningful results: silent meditation and slow breathing decelerate the action of the heart! Do we really need to go to India and study yogis in order to convince ourselves of that? Nor is the fact that deep meditation produces brain waves similar to those of dreamless sleep likely to shake the world.

Here again, the observation can do no more than establish that the adept is in a state of quietude. And any guru will tell you that that means nothing, that yoga is something else, in the physiological sphere as in others. What then? "This is what revelation teaches: through yoga one achieves total mastery over one's body; one is therefore able to modify it at will. A yogi can touch the moon with his fingers; he can make himself invisible; he understands the language of animals; he acquires the gift of second sight," etc. Of course, faithful as always to the scriptures, the gurus will also stress the triviality of these super-natural "powers," and remind you that the aim of yoga is salvation, not the performance of fairground stunts. But they will never deny the existence of the new powers acquired in this way. What is the Western observer to think when he hears a yogi say: "I have the gift of ubiquity; at this very moment I am at the same time conversing with you and with one of my disciples a thousand miles away," or when he is introduced to a person said to be two thousand years old? At best he can record the fact that such claims can be made, and accepted, within the cultural context of present-day Hinduism; nothing more, since it goes without saying that proof (either one way or the other) is impossible. And one feels only embarrassment when one reads about the simple-minded attempts of nineteenth-century British visitors to check "scientifically" the conditions under which such and such a yogi had himself buried alive (in order to "prove" that yoga conferred on him the power to survive with a minimum of oxygen), or to photo-graph the notorious Indian rope trick performed by fairground charlatans. It can be stated with confidence that if yoga's reputation had depended upon investigations of that kind, it would very quickly have vanished into oblivion!

It must therefore be conceded that any serious account of yoga must be based upon a reading of the normative texts and of what are gen-erally accepted as the authoritative commentaries on them, with direct observation occupying a useful secondary place, both as a means of checking that modern practice does in fact conform with the teachings of the masters of the past and as a way of evaluating any direct physical effects that yoga practices may possibly have upon the yogi's body. This book is based on those principles: it attempts to present a doctrinal synthesis of classical yoga backed up by observations on the "practical reality" of that doctrine. And this seems a good place to repeat for the last time that attempting to reduce yoga to any one of its multiple aspects (metaphysics, physical exercises, breath control, etc.) is seriously to mutilate it. When a Westerner unilaterally decides that the metaphysics of yoga does not interest him, that the physiology of the "vital breath" is just plain silly, but that "there is an element of validity in the breathing exercises and the postures," he is guilty of ideological imperialism—an error I intend to avoid in these pages. Nevertheless, as will become apparent later, I make no claim to be completely neutral in this matter. We all know today that total neutrality is not possible in the social sciences, since they form a domain in which the observer freely recognizes that his work is necessarily oriented and informed by his own subjectivity and must remain a function of the culture to which he belongs. So I shall simply say that yoga is presented here with sympathy (since otherwise I should never have undertaken this task), but also with a hint of Western skepticism, especially when it comes to describing the "miraculous powers" acquired by the yoga practitioner.

And if my reader, having closed this book, should feel a desire to know more about India, about dharma, about yoga, if he should then reopen the book and glance at the reading list at the back, as a prelude to continuing his inquiry into these cultural realities by which 450 million people live their lives but which are so little known among us, then I should not feel that a moment of the time I have spent writing it has been wasted.

Part 1

Man and the Universe

1. The Cosmic Order

raditional India knows that nothing in the universe is chance, that everything is necessity. In the infinite multiplicity of the real it reads a reference to unity, and perceives the rule of a sovereign order even where complexity seems in danger of lapsing into chaos and incoherence. The All, in itself and in each of its parts, is governed by an immutable, unbreakable law that supports the world while at the same time transcending it absolutely.

To this order, this law, the Hindu tradition gives the name *dharma,* a Sanskrit word with the primary meaning of maintenance, support, underpinning. The term appears as early as the Vedic period, even though it was not generally employed in its full meaning until the advent of classical Brahmanism.

The *Veda* in fact preferred the term *rita* to express the same idea. Rita, a verbal adjective, had the primary meaning of "fitted together," "ordered," and when used as a substantive denoted the universe itself. The importance of this semantic shift is clear: to the *rishis* (prophets, mythical authors of the Vedic poems), Someone (or Something) had, at the beginning of time, presided over the ordering of the world, had fitted it together. They said, for example, that a Great Architect had piled brick upon brick in order to build the cosmic house, just as a priest builds the altar of fire in order to celebrate a sacrifice. At other times the architect became a carpenter erecting a wooden temple, and at others the universe was compared to a chariot being assembled piece by piece by a divine cartwright.

Behind these images, the basic doctrine is clearly apparent: the world was constructed, not created ex nihilo; it was fabricated from preexisting elements that were assembled by an intelligence in such a way as to enable it to exist as an entity: bricks, beams, or planks were transformed, thanks to the intervention of that intelligence, into a dwelling, a temple, a vehicle. And to this organizing power the rishis sometimes gave the name Vishvakarman, the "Universal Craftsman,"

"He who has made all things," and conceived of him as an all-powerful deity emerging into activity in order to set the heaven and the earth in their places:

> *The god looks about on all sides,*
> *he turns to look in every direction;*
> *his hand acts everywhere, everywhere his foot!*
> *Working with his two arms,*
> *aided by the wings of his bellows,*[1]
> *he fits heaven and earth together,*
> *thereby bringing them into existence,*
> *the sole, the divine craftsman!*[2]

This kind of theology is not far removed from that found in the Bible (except that Vishvakarman only "fits together" the fragments of the universe, without first creating them out of chaos); but India would not be India if things were left as simple as that: in the same poem we find the question:

> *From what tree was it taken*
> *the wood he worked*
> *in order to construct heaven and earth?*
> *And on what did he take his stand*
> *when he raised the worlds into their places?*[3]

The important question here is not so much what the raw material was (the "tree" from which Vishvakarman took the wood for his beams) as what was taking the weight, what the support or foundation was. For the god must have had something to bear his weight while he undertook his creative labors, and the house he built could not have stood without firm footings. Here again the implications of the image are clear. The poem is saying that this demiurge is not in fact the all-powerful (since without something to take his weight he could not have constructed the worlds), and it suggests that the construction he has made is a precarious one (since it is dependent upon the earth in which its foundations are based).

There must therefore be something else, not only beyond the world (the house) but also beyond the creating god (the craftsman). And the *Upanishads* frequently designate this something else by the simple pronoun *tad* (That), which is a way of conveying that man has no possible way of expressing it adequately:

> *The something in which all things*
> *assemble and disperse,*
> *on which the gods have their seat,*
> *is That in the imperishable,*
> *the supreme firmament . . . .*
> *The something with which space*
> *and heaven and earth were filled,*
> *by whose means the sun warms,*
> *by whose means the waters generate life,*
> *is That: order and truth,*
> *the supreme brahman of the prophets!*
> *Navel of the universe,*
> *That sustains all things . . . .*[4]

The theological progress is clear: heaven, earth, the sun, the waters, the universe, put in their places by Vishvakarman, function by means of a mysterious power that "fills" them while also supporting them. This "foundation" is also the geographical location of all that exists, the point at which the constitutive elements of the cosmic machine "come together" (at the moment when the universal maker presides over the "creation" of the world) and "are dispersed" (when the world reaches its end). It is the navel of the universe, as the *Upanishad* poetically puts it. This power, this foundation, this mysterious location radically transcends phenomenal existence and is therefore situated beyond the perceptible in what the rishi terms "the imperishable, the supreme firmament": not Vishvakarman's paradise, but "a quite different world" of which man can say nothing.

Man has a need for words to communicate his intuitions, and that is why the "prophets" (rishis) sometimes resign themselves to giving a name to That which is nevertheless beyond the categories of name and form; at these times they call it *brahman*, as they called the beyond "the firmament." The word *brahman* came, after the *Veda*, to enjoy such vast prestige that Hinduism is sometimes referred to as Brahmanism, just as members of the highest caste are termed brahmins (in Sanskrit *brahmana*, "those who belong to brahman"). But the rishis nevertheless insisted indefatigably that brahman is not a person, not a god that can be venerated; at once transcendent and immanent, he or it is literally ungraspable and cannot therefore be the object of religious worship:

One cannot see him, one cannot grasp him; he has no family, no caste; he is without eyes, without ears, without hands, without feet; eternal, all-present, he penetrates all things; subtle, unalterable, he is the brahman, womb of all things, as the prophets know![5]

In other words, brahman is the Absolute, the principle on which everything depends, the cause of which the whole world is merely an effect, the essence of which existence is merely a phenomenon.

There might well have been the raw material here for a kind of metaphysical atheism. As God "of the philosophers and wise men," brahman could easily have been relegated (if one may so put it) to a beyond so distant that he would have retained hardly any more importance in men's eyes than the Voltairian deity of our eighteenth-century deists. However, the rishis did leave him with sufficient positive attributes to avoid that danger; by calling him "the womb of all things" (or "navel of the universe"), they were assimilating him, symbolically of course, to a human person, they were giving him a body. We must remember that a symbol, though of course the sign of a higher reality, is also a sign that speaks in the language of men; to say "womb" or "navel" is to evoke flesh to signify spirit, and both aspects of the symbol are equally valid and necessary.

Moreover, the symbol is never selected at random; in this instance it indicates that the Vedic rishis envisaged brahman as a man-cosmos, a *purusha* (the word means "male," then came to denote spirit forming a couple with the feminine *prakriti,* matter):

> *A thousand are the heads of the man-cosmos*
> *a thousand his eyes, a thousand his feet!*
> *He is all that is,*
> *all that was, all that will be. . . .*
> *From his navel the air came forth*
> *and from his head the heaven;*
> *the earth issued from his feet*
> *East and West from his ears:*
> *and that was how the world was formed![6]*

Later we shall see that this symbolic representation of brahman in the form of a man's body plays an important part in yoga doctrine. Here, however, we need only remember that classical Brahmanism is not far from making the Absolute into a sort of God the Father,

responsible for the construction of the universe (through the intermediary of his foreman, Vishvakarman or—as he is also called—
Prajapati, "Lord of creatures").

There are other positive values that are looked upon as representations ("incarnations") of brahman: the *Maha-Narayana Upanishad*
quoted earlier linked *tad* (That) with "order and truth" (*dharma* and
satya). In the same way, when asked by Pilate, "What is the Truth?"
Jesus answered, "I am the Truth." In other words, both the writer
of the Gospel and the rishis are telling us that the Absolute is also the
ultimate truth of all things. The world of phenomena would be no
more than a valueless illusion, a lie, if it were not the external, existential expression of an essential truth: Yahweh, brahman, the
Absolute.

But it is the notion of cosmic order (rita or dharma) that is given
the greatest emphasis in Hinduism and lends the whole religion its
specific color and originality. To say nothing of its name, since what
we call Hinduism is to Hindus *sanatana dharma,* "the eternal order."
The important thing here is that dharma is held to be an equivalent of
brahman, of the Absolute, not an expression of the divine will. When
the *Maha-Narayana Upanishad* tells us: "Dharma is the foundation of
the universe; yes it is upon It that the worlds are based, and it is It we
hold to be the sole support of all," it is stating as strongly as possible
the identity of That (the foundation, the cosmic support) with dharma.
It is therefore clear—contrary to an erroneous notion often expressed by
ill-informed Western writers—that the Hindu tradition is very far
from denying the world's reality. On the contrary, Hinduism attributes
the very highest reality to the world, since it makes it the material
expression of the Absolute. And not only that; dharma is at the same
time both matter and spirit, a union of the two principles by means of
which the universe is able to exist. And this "incarnation" of dharma,
forcefully revived by Tantrism, is a governing factor of one of yoga's
most important aspects, as we shall see later.

As well as being cosmic order and ultimate truth, dharma is also
the "essential reference," the "universal norm," the "law." As long
as we avoid giving any of these terms a moral significance, they can
be used to provide an adequate definition of Hinduism itself, inasmuch
as it claims to be an earthly, human embodiment of the Absolute. Not
that there are any statutes, any Ten Commandments, involved but,

rather, a sort of consensus enabling the cosmic machine to function: if the sun rises and sets at the proper time, that is dharma; if animals, men, and gods occupy their respective places in the chain of living beings, that is dharma; the fact that human beings all have their places in a hierarchy of castes, that they are divided into male and female and follow the biological cycle of birth, aging, and death, that too is dharma. Thus, evil to the Hindu, as you will probably have guessed, is anything that intervenes in any way in the life of the universe so as to disrupt it. For instance, the sun must rise at a given hour, and since dharma demands that men should offer up a sacrifice in order to cause the sun to rise, evil will be anything that involves a risk of that ritual act not being performed: idleness, illness, forgetfulness, impiety. Or it can also be the social decay that is leading brahmins to give their sons a Western-style education, one oblivious of the fact that the rhythm of the heavens is governed by sacrifice. For ignorance of this kind (and ignorance is probably the supreme evil since dharma is knowledge) spreads insidiously everywhere and saps the foundations of the cosmic house.

The world is not eternal. It is no more than one of dharma's possible forms, and like a living being it is born, develops, ages, dies. But dharma, being eternal, remains. Starting with the same materials as before, it constructs a new form, and so on through time, without there being any beginning or any end to this indefinite succession of universes: a tremendous vision which Hindu iconography usually represents symbolically in terms of a wheel (symbolized today on the Indian national flag) whose outer rim circles indefatigably and forever around its immutable axis (brahman). Dharma, in this image, is at once the axle, the hub, the movement, and lastly the whole wheel itself, inasmuch as it is an ordering separate elements held together as an entity solely by the fact that they constitute a wheel. The pieces of wood are nothing until the process of assembly that integrates them into a structure; and dharma is the structuring force, Spinoza's *natura naturans*. I must repeat here that this organizing energy is an intelligence, conscious of itself and taking delight in its work. Brahman (dharma) is *sach-chid-ananda,* "being-consciousness-joy," the *Upanishads* tell us, a statement that was used by certain medieval commentators, in particular Ramanuja,[7] as the foundation for a religion of *bhakti* (ardent devotion), and seen by others as an image of the Hindu trinity formed by the three gods Brahma (another name for Vishvakarman, the creator), Vishnu (the protector of the universe), and Shiva (responsible for the final dissolution of worlds that have reached the end of their allotted span).

These differences aside, however, all the Hindu masters agree in teaching that it is dharma, ever present at the center of the universe, that radiates like a spiritual sun the vivifying forces that enable it to come into existence in the first place and then to continue existing in the form laid down. I have already alluded to the existential multiplicity that blossoms or unfurls from the single principle, and here again the image of a wheel or a sun is used to make this clear: the "thousand beams" (rays or spokes) of both are symbolic of the complex (yet well-ordered) richness of the real in contrast to the naked simplicity of the single principle at the center. But here we meet a change in the imagery: the organization of the whole's innumerable parts, in accordance with dharma, takes a hierarchical form, and this leads to the image of a pyramid or mountain. The Hindus, resembling the Greeks in this respect, have their Olympus, which they call Meru and locate "at the center of the world" (which is to say, according to some traditions, at the North Pole). This mountain is not just the place where the gods live, it is first and foremost the world's axis (the hub of the cosmic wheel), and constitutes what might be termed a concretization of brahman (brahman "made perceptible to the eyes," to use the rishis' favorite phrase); from the mountain flow the four rivers that irrigate the world, upon it are fixed the sun and the moon, etc., as we are told in a famous poem from the *Atharva Veda* dedicated to the Cosmic Pillar (Mount Meru, brahman-axis of the world):

> *Taking his stand on the Pillar,*
> *Prajapati maintains the worlds.*
> *In his power he has the air and the earth,*
> *heaven, fire, the moon,*
> *the sun and the wind!*
> *Upon it are fixed the gods,*
> *the rishis, our ancestors,*
> *and the three Vedas.*
> *The Pillar supports the heaven,*
> *it upholds the earth, the atmosphere*
> *and the directions of space;*

men know this well
it is from the pillar that in the beginning
the gold of life spread through the world![8]

So we move imperceptibly from the image of the wheel, with brahman as its axis, to that of a universe organized as a pyramid.

The notion of diffusion, always present in the theology of brahman, implies in fact that things came into being successively. And this in turn means that their degree of participation in being is proportionate to their relative nearness to the single center, the parts farthest away being the heaviest (the coldest, the least animate, etc.), while the closer one comes to the central radiance, the more life, the more light, the more warmth one always finds. Similarly, the base of the mountain will be formed of the grossest cosmic elements, and as one climbs it so one finds progressively more and more subtle elements, until one reaches the summit which coincides with essence itself or, at the very least, with that form closest to essence. Seen from this point of view, dharma is the norm of reference that governs the position of all the constituent parts of the universe within the hierarchy: at the very bottom the most heavily material forms such as stones and the soil; at the very top the gods, whose existence is more "subtle" than that of any other kind of living being; and between these two extremes the unbroken chain of animal, human, "angelic," and divine species.

There is thus no break, no dialectical leap, no solution of continuity —simply a steady, imperceptible, upward progress from matter to spirit, even though it is permissible to classify the various categories of existence and to speak of various "worlds," a term that denotes different spheres of existence recalling the "aeons" of the Greek tradition. According to the authoritative texts of the Hindu tradition (*Upanishads, Bhagavad-Gita, Puranas*) there are three of these worlds: earth, atmosphere, and heaven. I must repeat, however, that these localizations are symbolic only; what they are primarily expressing is the relative distance of the beings inhabiting them from the source of life (here represented by the sun, or the eternal light shining above the celestial vault). The image of weight is also involved: earth is heavier than air, which is heavier in turn than the substance of heaven; and again there is the idea that the higher one goes, the richer, intenser, and happier life becomes. The implications of all this are manifold, but the general, underlying sense is clear enough.

Seen from this point of view, earth is the domain of those beings whose life is brutish and short: plant life, insects, mammals, men. Perpetually in search of food, condemned to constant effort, slaves of their instincts, all these beings are forever bowed beneath the law of necessity. Even within this domain, however, hierarchy still has its part to play. Stones, incapable of movement, of self-expression, are at the very bottom of the scale; above them are plants, already lighter, capable of autonomous movement, and living, like higher beings. After all, do they not come into being, develop, age, and die? And yet they also remain forever imprisoned in the earth by their roots and have little defense against external attacks ("the axe," the *Veda* says, "reigns as mistress over the forest). The decisive advantage of the animal kingdom is the faculty with which animals are endowed of moving about on the surface of the earth (or in the surface soil or the lower layers of the atmosphere). From the most fragile of insects to the largest and most awesome of wild beasts, the species of animal life reach up to the very limits of existence possible in the terrestrial world; and yet they still lack speech and the faculty of self-organization: monkeys and wolves can attain to the tribe, to the pack, but they never succeed in constructing a true society, and in that respect remain irremediably inferior to man.

Before considering man, however, I must emphasize that Hindus in no way despise the inferior forms of life. Very much the opposite: they hold that all life is sacred, whatever its form, since it is an expression of dharma, the cosmic law. Moreover, each of these forms is symbolic of some aspect of the universal order, which, as we have seen, is the same thing as the Absolute itself, brahman. This is why Hindus worship rocks, trees, and rivers and venerate animals. We all know, for example, that the cow is literally adored, even today, throughout the subcontinent; but the lion, the tiger, the monkey, the snake, etc., are no less so; and each animal species is also the living sign of one of the major deities: Vishnu's eagle, Shiva's cobra, Lakshmi's peacock, Ganesha's elephant, Agni's ram, Durga's tiger, and so on. Hence the rule of *ahimsa* (no injury to any living beings of whatever kind) which is given such prominence by many Hindu sects and of which, as we shall see, yoga makes one of the major virtues.[9]

Man stands at the very summit of the ladder of earthly beings; like the rest, he remains a prisoner of the limits inherent in this sphere of existence but he is also the only one of them endowed with freedom;

by using it he can transcend, to a considerable degree, his apparently animal condition (the physical differences between ape and man are minimal). Moreover, he is capable of metaphysical knowledge and therefore of knowing what dharma is (whereas the animals live dharma without knowing it)—a fact that enables him to organize his kind into societies constituted in the image of universal order; lastly, he has the power of articulate speech. This latter is important. Animals "talk," certainly, but the language they employ is purely mechanical, instinctive, and thus inadequate for conveying anything other than sensations: fear, hunger, sexual desire; whereas man, of course, has access to true language, the principal characteristic of which is that of being ordered or, in other words, of participating in dharma. This being so, it follows that there exists only one true language, the one that is called, appositely enough, *samskrita* (Sanskrit), a word that signifies "organized, normal, perfect." The gods, needless to say, speak only Sanskrit, and it is an indication of the eminent place man occupies in the creation that he possesses the privilege of being able to employ the divine tongue (*daivi vak*). As for the various languages or dialects that men speak in practice, the Brahmanic tradition regards all of them as merely bastardized derivatives of Sanskrit; and the fact that men can employ such debased tongues is one more sign of the decline of our present world.

Above earth, but below heaven, there lies an intermediate region that is symbolically referred to as the atmosphere. This is the aerial domain of a vast number of living beings whose physical and mental capacities are superior to those of all terrestrial beings while still falling short of those enjoyed by the inhabitants of heaven. These beings are normally invisible to men, because they do not belong to the same sphere of existence; but they do possess the power of visiting the earth, if they so wish, and appearing to humans or to animals. The Brahmanic tradition distinguishes a great many categories of genies, angels, demons, nymphs, vampires, dragons, etc., all of which share a number of characteristics specific to what one might call the denizens of the in-between (between men and gods): longevity, ability to move through space "as swiftly as lightning," magic powers (increasing or decreasing their size at will, producing fantasms, knowing the past and future, etc.).

Among the most important of these beings (that is, among those who tend to intervene in human affairs) are the Gandharvas, who

inspire musicians, singers, and dancers; they may on occasion take over
a human ("from within") and lead him to behave in bizarre ways; nor
do they scorn the pleasure of seducing women. The Apsaras are the
Indian nymphs; habitual companions of the Gandharvas, they take
great pleasure in disturbing men's minds by inspiring them with "the
madness of love"; they are also responsible for men's passion for
gambling, and for stirring up the madness of war: after a battle is
over they come down and select their lovers from among the warriors
who have fallen in the fight. The Rakshasas (guardians) possess
distinctly demoniac characteristics: they torment men by dazzling their
eyes with the gold and precious stones of their secret treasures. The
vampires (Pishachas) haunt cremation sites looking for unburned
corpses they can inhabit in order to terrorize the living. The Nagas are
much like dragons, and as ambivalent in their attitude: they protect
those they love but are fearful foes to those who displease them.

All this must not be allowed to give us a false impression, however;
these angels, demons, and genies all have lives of their own to live
quite independently of mankind. It is natural that men should be
particularly interested in adventures that involve contact with the
inhabitants of the world above theirs, but such meetings form only a
small part of the genies' lives. The Brahmanic tradition tells us that
their sphere of existence is as abundantly peopled as our own: Gandharvas, Apsaras, and Rakshasas all live in aerial cities built of crystal,
gold, and diamond, floating in the air like Rimbaud's "cloud cathe-
drals." The life of feasts and pleasures they lead in them bears a
strong resemblance to the paradisaic delights that occupy the dreams of
the pious looking forward to their rewards after death; but it still
remains distinctly inferior to the beatitude enjoyed by the gods.

These latter, of course, are the occupants of the third sphere of
existence—heaven. The name is used to denote this higher world in a
symbolic fashion only, as is made quite clear by the fact that the Hindu
tradition describes such and such a god as living in the Himalayas,
another in the sea, another beneath the earth. So the name "heaven" is
simply an image intended to convey that the gods are "above" all other
beings, and that their specific domain is that of the light that radiates
from the vault of heaven. In that high region, where the stars, the
sun, and the moon have their motion, existence can only be joy, warmth,
freedom; it is the most beautiful form that life can take, at least while
still remaining separate from brahman (which of course absolutely

transcends all forms of existence). Heaven, like earth and atmosphere, is peopled by an infinite number of living beings; Hinduism is a perfect polytheism.

Even in heaven, however, since it too is an integral part of the universe, there is a hierarchy, an organization obeying the laws of dharma. Occupying the lowest rung of the celestial ladder we find the divine troops or bands (*gana*) whose innumerable members are scarcely to be distinguished from the angels and genies of the atmospheric space sphere. These minor gods constitute the courts as it were, of the more important gods, whom they assist in their cosmic functions.[10] Indra, for example, who presides over the cosmic order's more violent manifestations (wars against the forces of evil, storms and tempests, etc.), is habitually accompanied by his band of Maruts, young warriors whose arms glitter like the lightning flash. Yama, god of death, sends down his messengers when a living being reaches the end of its span of existence; their task is to carry away its soul to the underground place where it will be judged. Varuna, guardian of the universal law, employs "spies" who keep a ceaseless watch on the behavior of every living being. The possible examples are legion, and in some cases these divine bands have a leader whose duty is to act as intermediary between the servant group and their Lord. We find Shiva, for example, delegating his powers to an intermediate deity (inferior to him but superior to those who obey his orders) to whom tradition simply gives the name Ganapati[11] (leader of the troops) or Ganesha.

Above these hordes of divine subordinates, the more important gods themselves are also divided into great bands, which might be called tribes or clans, standing more or less in a state of vassalage to the three cosmic sovereigns Brahma, Vishnu, and Shiva. Among the most important of these clans we find the Vasus (presiding over the elements and vital forces), the Rudras (whose function is to keep alive the various forms of energy that constitute the universe), the Adityas (sons of Aditi, Freedom; they are responsible for the cosmic "virtues" such as the strict observance of dharma, the law of hospitality, generosity, the vital impulse, etc.).

There are many other groups besides these, even if we leave aside the "solitary" gods, notably those embodying the principal forces at work in the universe: Agni (Fire), Apas (the Waters), Surya (Light), and so on. And finally, at the very summit of the divine hierarchy, we find enthroned the three sovereign beings who together constitute the Hindu trinity (*trimurti*, "the three divine forms"): Brahma (not to be confused with brahman, the Absolute), Vishnu, and Shiva. The first fulfills the role of demiurge: when a cosmic cycle comes to an end, when the constituent elements of the universe have been dissociated and matter (prakriti) has returned to chaos, then Brahma forms dharma into a new reality by organizing matter once more and thus giving birth to another universe. This new universe which must be created, since the world (being eternal) cannot not exist, is always the same (because all matter is one) yet always different (because the possibilities involved in the assembly process are infinite in number). In Nietzsche's phrase: "It is always the same world but it is always different." His role fulfilled, Brahma then withdraws (or goes to sleep, according to some).

Vishnu's role is to ensure the preservation of the universe that Brahma has "created." To Vishnu, therefore, falls the task of safeguarding dharma, which also entails the functions of judgment (reward for the virtuous, punishment for the wicked). From this point of view he is certainly the Hindu deity most nearly resembling the god of the Bible—especially since Vishnu, like God the Father of the Gospels, also incarnates himself in order to save the world when it is in danger. However, India is too fond of multiplicity to restrict herself to a single "Son": Vishnu "descends" on numerous occasions, and in each case assumes a form appropriate to the circumstances. Among the most important of these "descents" (*avatara*—hence our word "avatar") are the following examples: in order to save the last of the righteous at the time of the great flood, Vishnu took the form of a fish that guided Manu's ark to the one mountain spared by the waters;[12] when the earth was almost carried down by the Evil One into the depths of the cosmic ocean, Vishnu became a boar and brought it back up to the surface; on another occasion he became a lion in order to tear a demon apart; and so forth.

The list of such "descents" is a long one, but probably the one that exceeds all the others in popularity in India itself is that in which Vishnu incarnated himself as Krishna. Taking the form of a man this time (as he had already done before when incarnated as Rama), he took upon himself the man's total destiny, from birth to death, with the purpose of helping mankind to surmount the crisis inaugurating the entry of this particular world into its Kali-Yuga.[13] In the great battle waged on the Kurukshetra (not far from present-day Delhi), Krishna intervened as the inspirer and guide of Prince Arjuna, the champion of dharma. The famous text of the *Bhagavad-Gita* contains the instructions Krishna gave to Arjuna just before battle was joined: the god reminds him in the strongest terms that during the perilous era of the Kali-Yuga men's salvation is only possible through a strict observance of the cosmic law with the help of God (Vishnu-Krishna). Other legends, retold in many devotional works, deal with other moments in Krishna's life; in particular there is the story of how, as an adolescent, the young prince wooed the village milkmaids; how he played tricks on his mother as a child; and how his sovereign power manifested itself even when he was still in the cradle. All these stories agree in presenting Krishna as a familiar and very human incarnation. This image of him provided the foundation for the devotional movement that left so deep an imprint upon popular Hinduism.

Shiva, for his part, will preside over the dissolution of the world when it reaches the end of its allotted span (an event that according to Hindu tradition cannot now be long delayed). However, the god does not remain inactive during the duration of the cosmic cycle. He too can intervene to save the world if the appropriate time for its dissolution has not yet arrived, as he did, for example, when he swallowed the poison that was threatening to corrupt its primal matter. And although he does not strictly speaking incarnate himself as Vishnu does, he nevertheless has sons who act in his name and intervene under his direction in the affairs of the universe. All forms of violence (provided it is necessary and salutary) fall within his domain. This may mean encouraging the use of the martial virtues at times when cowardice would permit the Evil One to triumph; it may also mean love in its aggressive forms (for if the Indian Eros, Shiva's son, carries a bow, it is in order to transfix the hearts of lovers with his darts in good earnest); or it may mean death, which is beneficial to the righteous since it enables them to ascend to paradise. The intellectual obstacles put in men's ways by his son Ganapati (or Ganesha) are likewise a blessing from Shiva, since they enable the deserving to demonstrate their abilities.

In consequence, as we shall see later, Shiva is the patron of all yogis, precisely because yoga is an arduous undertaking, a path strewn with obstacles and that demands heroic fortitude on the part of the adept who follows it. Salvation is achieved through Shiva, since he it is who sets the difficulties in the way, while at the same time providing the graces that will enable them to be overcome (though only faithful disciples are able to benefit from them). And yoga apart, Shiva is also man's guide in any undertaking directed toward salvation, which is why he is so often represented in Hindu iconography as a naked ascetic, covered in ashes as a sign of penitence (whereas Vishnu is bedecked with jewels and clothed in precious stuffs). And in his hair Shiva wears a crescent moon, because the powers of the night also belong to him (whereas Vishnu is a solar deity). Sometimes too he is venerated in the form of a dancer juggling with fire: each of the flames he holds in the air is a universe Shiva has destroyed at the moment required by dharma; and together they form a circle of fire symbolizing the permanence of matter through all the multiple forms it infinitely assumes.

This presentation of the hierarchic Hindu universe, ordered in accordance with the laws of dharma, would not be complete if we omitted to point out that at every level we have mentioned the forces in question are in fact double, since in each case one can discern both a male and a female element. Life, for example, is a permanent union of water and fire, dry and wet, day and night, etc. And water is in fact a female element (wet, nocturnal, lunar) that is fertilized by fire, a male element (dry, diurnal, solar). Living beings are likewise divided into the two sexes (since everything dependent upon dharma must also present all the characteristics of dharma), from the insects right up to the highest divinities. So there is no god not assisted by his consort: Sarasvati, goddess of creative intelligence, is the wife of Brahma; Lakshmi, goddess of fortune, beauty, and prosperity, is the wife of Vishnu; Parvati ("the mountain goddess") is the wife of Shiva.[14] It will have become apparent by now that consorts of the gods are as it were a divine representation of the essential functions assumed by their husbands: since Vishnu presides over the happy conservation of dharma, it is fitting that Lakshmi should be the distributor of wealth.

This polarity is evident on every level of existence. For instance, the Apsaras are the partners of the Gandharvas in the intermediate sphere, just as women are the partners of men on earth. And as you may have guessed, this fundamental dualism (which is not entirely unlike the opposition between *yin* and *yang* in the Chinese tradition) plays a decisive role in the theory and practice of yoga.

2. Man as Analogue

The evocation of dharma, in the preceding pages, as cosmic order was by no means irrelevant to our purpose. It was intended not merely to gratify the reader's curiosity but to open a door for him into the yogi's mental universe. The notion of hierarchical planes of existence occupies a central position in the doctrine since everything in it is based upon the idea of spiritual progress, of a gradual ascent toward the higher forms of existence. And such progress, such a "climb to Carmel," in the words of Saint John of the Cross, also implies some kind of correspondence between the cosmic order and the organization of the human individual since otherwise the very notion of such an ascent might prove groundless. The existence of such a correspondence is, in fact, precisely what traditional Brahmanism has been teaching persistently for five thousand years, from the *Veda* to Ramakrishna and Aurobindo:[1] not only is there no break in continuity anywhere in the chain of existential forms, but also, and above all, each link in that chain is formed in the image of the whole, just as the whole is in the image of each of its parts.

Hinduism, like the Hermetic tradition, inclines to believe that "what is below is like what is above"; so that the man who knows how to use his eyes is able to see dharma in all things, and thus to behave in conformity with the eternal norm, which is always and everywhere present. This adherence to the principle of analogy governs all the processes of Indian thought. It is the basis upon which all Hindu doctrinal edifices are built, whatever divergences may occur between the various schools on other points. And naturally, although this principle operates at all levels, it is with its operation on the human plane that we humans are mainly concerned. It is in fact twofold: on the one hand every individual is a universe in miniature, a complete and faithful image of the entire cosmos; on the other, the human community as a whole is, in its organization, an incarnation of cosmic dharma—the organizing power of total reality.

Indeed, as we have already seen, it is impossible for Brahmanism to conceive of anything happening by chance or by a simple interplay of fortuitous contingencies, since it is fundamental to the tradition that everything that exists bears witness—both in itself and in its relation to every other form of existence—to the eternal order of the cosmos. It is therefore unthinkable to regard human society as being one possible society among others. In the eyes of Indian tradition, the relations of men to other men are determined neither by a conjunction of historical circumstances nor by freedom; they are regulated by the universal law. Or, rather, they are the normal expression of that law. This granted, humanity must necessarily present the same characteristics as the cosmos, since it is a sort of tracing or copy of it. Which, in turn, means that human society must be hierarchized in the same way as the entire chain of living beings, from insects to gods.

The social expression of this hierarchy is of course the caste system, one of the most strikingly original facets of Indian society.[2] The principle behind it is well known: men are in no way equal one to another (either in natural fact or in law). Just as the animal order is divided into species, so humans too are divided into distinct groups. Just as a wolf and a lamb are both animals but differ profoundly in their behavior—and also, one might add, as to the final purpose of their existence within the animal kingdom—so a brahmin and a pariah, while both are men, belong in fact to different social categories possessing neither the same rights nor the same duties (although both are contributing to the human sphere's expression of universal harmony).

In order that dharma may effectively regulate human society, it is thus necessary for this society to be organized into groups and subgroups, at once autonomous and interdependent, which together constitute what is called in Sanskrit the *dharma-rajya,* a term that might be rendered by "normal society" (that is, conforming to the norm, to dharma). In this ideal system all individuals belong, from birth, to a multitude (several hundred) of autonomous communities that are known to Indians as *jatis* (births) and to us as "castes," the name given to them by the Portuguese when they described them for the first time in the sixteenth century. These jatis are arranged hierarchically, and it is once again the pyramid (or cosmic mountain) image that is predominant: the lower castes are also the most massive numerically, those that provide the largest contingent of individuals while the higher castes contain a relatively smaller number. And tradition, repeating what it says about the organization of living beings in the universe, justifies this inequality with the theory of relative distances from being-in-itself (brahman): the human beings farthest from the essential light have their place in the shadowy provinces; those who are nearest to it (still within the sphere of existence specific to men, i.e., the earth) inhabit the peak of the mountain, so that it is not without good reason that they are named brahmins. This light symbolism derives, it will be remembered, from that other image of the universe as a solar wheel illumined by the beams of brahman, its hub, the world axis. Tradition, when viewing the universe in these terms, says that it is the relative distance between any being and the luminous source that determines to which one of the three cosmic categories—*tamas* (darkness or shadow), *rajas* (energy), or *sattva* (conformity with being)—that being shall belong. And this threefold division of the levels of existence in terms of their "cosmic qualities" *(gunas)* is yet one more instance of the Indian passion for trinitarian groupings.[3] I need hardly specify that on the cosmic level it is the earth that comes under the head of tamas, the atmosphere under that of rapas, and heaven under that of sattva.

On the human level, this theory of cosmic qualities makes it possible to impose an order upon the teeming multiplicity of jatis. Employing the symbolism of color, which attributes black to the tamas, red to the rajas, white to the sattva, the castes or jatis are divided into three broad functions termed *varnas* (colors). This means that one can recognize the place of each jati in the social pyramid by its appropriate color, it being understood that we are dealing here with shades of light, variations in intensity, rather than with colors in the proper sense of the term: red gives off more light than black, but less than white. The varnas—and this must be stressed, if only because some people have thought they could be construed as vestiges of racial differences—are nothing more than a visual metaphor intended to indicate the hierarchy of the broad caste groups by reference to their respective distances from the eternal brahman-light.

These three broad functions divide human labor into production of wealth, the exercise of violence, and spiritual authority. In Sanskrit, the individuals belonging to the three varnas are *vaishyas* (producers, merchants, clerks), or *kshatriyas* (those exercising executive power, from police constables to kings), or *brahmanas* (intellectuals, priests, magicians—here called "brahmins"). The same type of division is to be found in all the Indo-European peoples, particularly, as the work of Georges Dumézil has shown,[4] among the Latins, Celts, Germans, and Slavs; nor is there any cause for surprise here, since we know that the essentials of Indian civilization were derived from the Aryans who established themselves in the northwest part of the subcontinent during the third and second millennia B.C.[5] It is nevertheless true that Hinduism stamped the mark of its own genius upon the ideology of the three functions by putting a tremendous emphasis on hierarchy (whereas Rome, for example, effectively abolished it) and by developing the metaphysical theory justifying this hierarchy from the doctrine of relative distance between the levels of existence and the essential principle.

Side by side with this theoretical division into the three varnas, another partition in effect separated society into two "camps": that of the holders of power (brahmins and kshatriyas) and that of the producers. In the *Veda* we find perpetual praise of the two forces (*ubhe viriye*) that govern the world: spiritual authority and temporal power. Numerous famous passages explain that the one is nothing without the other and that together they are invincible; and entire philosophy is built up around the theory of the relationship between the king (kshatriya par excellence) and his chaplain (*purohita,* prototype of the brahmins). But this harmonious dialectic does not succeed in concealing the historical reality of the clergy-nobility conflict.

We know that among most of the Indo-European peoples of antiquity (principally in Rome, Greece, and among the Teutons) the kshatriyas succeeded in relegating the brahmins to secondary status; in India, on the contrary, the triumph of the first function was total: not only was Indian culture completely brahminized (that is to say, it accepted the values specific to the brahmin caste as universal laws), but those jatis belonging to the second function vanished almost completely. This "evaporation" of an entire (or almost entire) varna is very strange. Lacking precise historical evidence as we do, it has been conjectured that a fair number of families were physically eliminated during the troubled centuries just before and just after the beginning of the Christian era, when India was subject to invasions and internal wars that ravaged her northern and western provinces. Then, later, there were the Moslems with their ruthless determination to destroy the Hindu nobility. But the primary cause is thought to be the fact that the kshatriya families all systematically tried to marry their children to brahmins, in order to raise themselves gradually to what they took to be a higher social position. And lastly, from the tenth century onward, it became increasingly in the kshatriyas' interest to be converted to Islam, since that was their only way to preserve political power over their fiefs now that they were vassals of the Moslem rulers.

For centuries, then, the theory of three varnas has failed to correspond to observable reality. The actual situation, both in classical (since the fifth century after Christ) and in modern India, is one of continuous conflict between the many jatis of what we might call the third estate and the few *gotras* or brahmin clans. The vaishyas, the brahmins, and the very few kshatriyas still surviving, if taken all together, now constitute the entire population of "high-caste Hindus," and they are the only members of the population who play an important role in the various sectors of Indian culture— the only ones who, as the scriptures put it, "may speak in the name of dharma." Yet this group contains barely half of India's Hindu population, the remaining half comprising the tens of millions of outcastes.

The very oldest tradition did in fact recognize the existence of these people, whom it called *shudras,* and there are some texts that even go so far as to speak of a fourth varna, to which they belonged. But such a position is not really tenable, since it destroys the doctrinal edifice based upon the analogy between the three functions and the three cosmic qualities (and what fourth color could we find that would be darker than the black of *tamas,* the shadows?). The real social situation remains the opposition between the twice-born (*dvijas*)—so called because they alone are admitted to the ritual ceremony of institution (*upanayana*)[6]—and all other Hindus: shudras and pariahs.

Hierarchic distinctions can of course be made among the broad mass of "lower" humans too. Thus at the very summit of this group one would place the shudras proper (those theoretically exercising functions of service), and at the very bottom the pariahs (*chandalas*), sometimes referred to as "untouchables" because contact with them, even by chance, entails ritual defilement for the "twice-born," who must then purify themselves by means of specific ceremonies codified in the "Manuals of Dharma."[7] The Brahmanic tradition itself does not pay much attention to these distinctions, however; in its eyes, the outcastes remain an undifferentiated mass of beings placed by their birth outside the norm (dharma).

Yet their very existence poses a theological problem, since it is evident that if the universe were in fact regulated by dharma, there would only be three broad groups of humans, just as there are only three worlds (heaven, atmosphere, earth), three cosmic qualities (sattva, rajas, tamas), three sovereign gods (Brahma, Vishnu, Shiva), and so on. The reply to this is that the present situation of humanity is a "sign of the times": we are now in the final cosmic age, Kali-Yuga, in which we see the influence of dharma shrinking back into itself like Balzac's *Peau de Chagrin.* The number of those with access to the Brahmanic rites (and thus meriting the title *dvijas*) is constantly diminishing, relatively at least; those of mankind furthest from the heart of the earth[8] are progressively (but in accordance with a "negative progression" that is in fact regression) "forgetting" dharma, and as the light emanating from the sacred center fades, so the influence of tamas (the "cosmic quality" of the shadows) lengthens across the world.

This explains how the inhabitants of the five continents became "barbarians" (*mlecchas*). Then the evil attacked India itself, in the form of intercaste marriages that destroyed the natural order, and, having fallen from the position guaranteed by their former religious rights, the children of these irregular unions gradually built up the new category of outcastes. This "barbarization" of Indian society is constantly accelerating if we are to believe the tradition: have we not seen men born Hindus reject the religion of their fathers and go over to Buddhism, to Islam, to Christianity? And finally, in our own day, it is the very principle of a society instituted in conformity with dharma that has been contested, since the constitution of the Republic of India stipulates—since 1949— that any reference to the caste system is forbidden by law. Orthodox Hindus conclude from this that the world has now moved into the darkest days of the Kali-Yuga.

The fact that the appearance of the "outcaste" category has been attributed to intercaste marriages is significant in that it enables us to understand how the system works. The high-caste Hindu belongs by birth to a particular jati comprising a larger or smaller number of family clans all occupying the same social rank. And it is exclusively within the framework of this community that the individual must live his religious life: the rites celebrated on the occasion of his birth, then at his initiation, his marriage, the birth of his own children, and his death, must all bear public witness to his membership of a given caste.

In consequence, it is unimaginable that he would marry outside that caste, a fact that reduces freedom of choice for would-be bridegrooms to a minimum.

In practice, however, marriages are for the most part arranged by the parents, in accordance with the demands of family expediency (material interests) or of religion (they consult priests or astrologers or both). Frequently the betrothed couple do not even see one another for the first time until their wedding day.[9] Since the sole function of marriage is the perpetuation of the family (and therefore of the jati), there can be no grounds for permitting feelings to interfere in what in the eyes of tradition is merely the performance of a duty. Love exists in India, of course, as it does everywhere, but it arises between bride and groom only after marriage[10] or, more often, seeks its freedom in adultery. The stories told of Krishna are significant in this respect. We see him not only seducing the village milkmaids (even though they are married) but also neglecting his legitimate wife Rukmini while granting his favors to his mistress Radha,[11] and yet both rustic dalliance and extramarital love affair are presented as examples of perfect love symbolizing the felicity of the soul receiving the gift of grace from its Lord.

The other caste obligation concerns commensality: the Hindu is strictly forbidden to take meals with anyone belonging to a lower caste, or to eat food prepared by "impure" hands (that is, by a cook not of the same caste or a higher one). Since these principles apply to all dvijas, it will be appreciated that, in practice, the orthodox Hindu can eat no dishes other than those prepared for him by his wife.

Such rules may sometimes have unexpected consequences. For example, brahmins have proved quite ready to hire themselves out as cooks, and are consequently very much in demand as such by rich vaishyas. For although it would be infringing the law to eat food prepared by an inferior, there is no danger of doing so when eating meals cooked by a superior. Moreover, the superior is not committing any sin if he cooks vegetables for an inferior. On the other hand, a brahmin may not sit at the table of a vaishya (or receive him into his house), since the mere fact of eating together would involve a defilement of superior by inferior. Which is why meals in India can never become the social functions they so often are in the West. The Hindu either eats alone or with his peers, and even in the latter case there is still a rule that the meal should be taken in silence, since the consumption of food is a liturgical ceremony, a rite requiring meditation for its performance. Even married couples do not take their meals together; the wife serves her husband (and her sons after they have received their initiation) and then eats what is left, after he has finished, in the kitchen. And let us not forget that, until not long ago, this was still customary in some rural areas of Europe.

It will have been noticed that the "sanction" entailed by any infringement of dharma is of an exclusively religious kind: the brahmin who accepts food offered by a pariah (to take the most extreme example) is defiled by that act; but the impurity is operative only on the ritual level: it merely entails the impossibility of fulfilling the required daily religious observances. In order to cleanse oneself from the impurity, one must do penance (for example, fasting for some longer or shorter period, bathing in holy water, in a sacred river or pool, making an offering in the temple). These expiations are clearly proportionate to the degree of the error committed, which is to say, to the hierarchic distance separating tainter from tainted: the brahmin lives in fear of exposing himself to the danger of a chance contact (intention has no bearing, since the error exists only as a concrete fact), whereas the lowest jatis run much less danger since they can be tainted only by untouchables.

The expiations required may seem somewhat lacking in severity, since even those laid down for major infringements consist merely in fasting, and quite often the fast is less than absolute, as is shown by this prescription from the *Manava-Dharma-Shastra*, 11.152:

> *He who eats food*
> *prepared by people of a lower caste*
> *or leavings from a woman's meal*
> *must eat only boiled barley*
> *for seven days and seven nights.*

But it is a well known fact that penance is never intended to be penal in character in the majority of religions; it is meant only as a sign of repentance carrying the promise of redemption. Hinduism is no exception; it heals its practitioners of the consequences of an act of a similar nature. The error was ritual, and so the expiation is ritual too; but, in a society ruled by dharma, nothing can be more important than rites, since they are the very workings of dharma conceived of as an enduring cosmic liturgy. Every error disrupts the universal harmony and contributes to the degradation of the conditions of our world's existence: the fact that we live in the Kali-Yuga is at once a consequence of the lapses for which we are daily responsible toward dharma and also the cause of those errors (since the world's progress toward its own end is ineluctable). The important thing is that we as individuals should be painfully aware of those lapses, take the fault of them upon ourselves, and make haste to expiate them.

India is still a profoundly religious country. It is almost impossible to find a dvija who does not scrupulously observe his caste duties and, more particularly, his ritual obligations. Morning and evening prayers, veneration of the divinities that stand on the small family altar, observance of the liturgical feasts, participation in pilgrimages, ablution in sacred water sources, fasts at the times fixed by caste tradition—nothing is omitted by the heads of families, who are always fully supported by the women and children of the household. These fascinating ceremonies, easily observable by outsiders once the trust of the family has been gained, lend a particular color to contemporary Indian society, which is still faithful in these matters to the legacy of the Ancients; and the Western travelers who have been struck by this fact are legion.

This being so, it is easy to understand why infringements of caste rules are experienced as a serious matter by those who have committed them or who have been witness to them. We must not forget that such errors are, by definition, public, since they require the presence of at least two persons—defiler and defiled. Moreover, privacy does not exist in India, and nothing is secret; each individual lives and goes about his business in the light of common day, surrounded by kinfolk from whose eyes nothing he does can possibly be hidden. Even in the very rare case of a person who himself feels no concern for religious matters, social pressure (and first and foremost family pressure) are such that he cannot avoid doing penance if he commits an infringement.

However, it must be emphasized that there can be no question of coercion exercised by any kind of external authority (police or family council). Infringements of dharma relate exclusively to the metaphysical plane, and the civil laws are concerned only with punishing crimes against society, so that the penalties they inflict play no role in the religious sphere. The thief is defiled by his action (since it is contrary to dharma), and he will remain tainted, even after serving a prison sentence, until he has done penance in accordance with the rules of his caste. And inversely, a ritual expiation, however harsh, does not preclude a penal sanction imposed by society. This does not mean that in certain cases, where there is room for dispute, a group of elders may not constitute themselves into a "caste court" in order to determine what particular expiation a particular offender should undergo.

It is for this reason that the Sanskrit literature includes a large number of *Dharma-Shastras* (Manuals of Dharma) which sometimes contradict one another; though it must be clearly understood that such contradictions will always concern points of detail only (length of fast prescribed, for example), never the doctrine itself, upon which all are in agreement: that man is analogous to the universe and that he belongs in consequence, "by natural law," to a hierarchized society in the image of the cosmos.

We should add that the average Hindu experiences his jati, the caste to which he belongs, as a supportive structure that protects him and provides him with a very strong sense of security, in contrast to the egalitarian society, which throws the individual very much upon his own resources. Everything in India contributes to this integration of the individual into an order that is recognized as being transcendent (because it is dharma): the family has not been reduced to the nuclear form so familiar to us; instead, it spreads out to include collateral relatives, parents, and grandparents. The result is a group of dozens of individuals all conforming to a precisely laid down hierarchy of precedence and all with their part to play in the management of the family estate (which cannot legally be divided). Each person's place is marked out in advance upon this family chessboard, as it were, and the sense of security engendered by such a life style is not hard to understand; parents, wives, children, all live with the assurance of never being abandoned, of being cared for throughout their lives by the family community. So their entire time on earth is spent within a microcosm of the universe in which they are consciously fulfilling a role to which they were destined even before their birth.

A woman, for example, must be "guarded" (i.e., protected, fed) by her father while she is a child, by her husband when she is an adult, by her sons when she is old and widowed.[12] And if by some ill chance her husband were to disappear before her sons were old enough to protect her, then that role would be assumed by her husband's brothers. The Manuals of Dharma lay down in the minutest detail the line of conduct to be followed in every imaginable case. What is to be done, for example, if the bridegroom dies before the wedding? The *Manava-*

Dharma-Shastra replies: "If the husband-to-be dies before the ceremony, then his brother shall take the bride-to-be with him and visit her
regularly until she has conceived."[13] And there is a good reason for
this. Since the sole purpose of marriage is the propagation of the species
(and in India that means patrilinear descent), it is essential that the
wife should give birth to a son who will belong to her husband's family,
even if that husband should himself happen to become unavailable
before he has had time to engender it.

This gives some idea of the detail the Manuals of Dharma are
prepared to go into in laying down rules of behavior. But what I am
really concerned with here is not the exploration of these sometimes
curious details of the behavioral code but rather a demonstration of the
extent to which all Hindus' lives are determined by their social situation. For we must not forget that, extending beyond the family, is the
caste, which is a kind of federation of family clans all occupying the
same social stratum, and one more framework into which the external
activities of the family's active members must be inserted.[14] Then,
beyond the groups of families, the individual recognizes the varna to
which his caste belongs. Taking a broader view still, he will also have
a strong emotional awareness of his membership in the Hindu community (as opposed to other Indian communities—the Moslems, the
Christians, etc.). This tight network of social relationships keeps each
individual firmly in place and helps him to live out his life as dharma.
Thus the hierarchic structure of the universe, the principle of analogy,
the concept of cosmic order, the opposition between single essence and
the multiplicity of existence are not abstract ideas to the Hindu. They
are concrete realities, of which his religious instruction simply helps
him to become aware; which is probably why Hinduism remains the
dynamic force it is, even today.

3. Sarvam Duhkham

conception of the universe as a perfectly organized Whole, the knowledge that all living beings, both in their internal structure and their external relations, are analogous with the world of which they are part, the belief that there is a cosmic intelligence keeping watch over the order of things and, moreover, embodied by that order—all this ought to provide grounds for metaphysical and religious optimism, for a luminous, serene ideology. Yet the first Westerners who gained access to Hinduism's fundamental texts were struck by the pessimism expressed in them.[1] To restrict ourselves to yoga itself, it is significant to find in the *Yoga-Sutras,* the basic text of the doctrine, Patanjali exclaiming: *Duhkham eva sarvam vivekinah* ("For those who know, all is merely pain"). And this is not just a sort of cynical proverb on the lines of "Vanity of vanities" from *Ecclesiastes.* The terms employed by the rishi go deeper than that, because *sarvam* (the whole) was in fact the word then currently in use to denote the universe in its totality, and *duhkham* (pain) means not just "suffering, misfortune" but first and foremost evil-in-itself, in whatever forms it attempts to disguise itself (even if those forms are pleasure, the joys of life, the magic of nature). Thus, Patanjali is ultimately saying that evil is everywhere, that it exists in all things, that it manifests itself in the form of universal suffering. But how is one to reconcile such a position (adopted, we must remember, by all the Hindu doctrinal texts, however diverse the deductions that may subsequently be drawn from them) with the doctrine of dharma? After all, if it is true that all things are in the image of the sovereign good, how can it be claimed at the same time that they are identical with evil?

To Hindu thinkers, the paradox is only on the surface. Nature, in their eyes, is so beautiful that they call it *maya* (magic).[2] As aware as anyone of the glamor of life's multiple, dynamic, outward forms, they could well say with the psalmist that the skies "proclaim the glory of God." Ecstatic religious experience is often compared in Hindu scrip-

41

ture to the intuition of beauty; it may be written, for example, that the mystic vision of brahman is like the cry of a man seeing a white bird flying before the black clouds of the monsoon. Love, our daily joys on earth, are so many "proofs" that the world refers ultimately to dharma. And such experiences, of course, are not the exclusive prerogative of man; they exist among the animals and increase in number as one ascends the scale of beings. The Gandharvas and the Apsaras suffer less than we do from the necessities of life (they live longer, they do not grow old); the gods are wholly ignorant of them: they suffer no corporeal limitations or distress; it is said of them, significantly, that they walk without needing to touch the earth with their feet, and that they see without ever needing to blink.

Not only this, but the ordering of the universe is in itself a manifestation of beauty and intelligence; Hindus compare it to a *mandala* (circle; see figure 7). As we know, this kind of symbolic design, made up of simple geometric figures (squares, triangles, circles), drawn on the ground with colored sand or painted on cloth, is used by gurus to evoke a direct intuition of the cosmic order in their disciples by making them absorb its abstract perfection. That the world is beautiful (and therefore good) is self-evident. And to know as much is happiness. No Hindu would contradict that; but the master's duty is to lead his disciples beyond the magic, beyond the multiple glamors of maya. To this end, he will begin by forcing him into an awareness of beauty's fragility. That young body in which all is harmonious grace, is it not doomed by nature to wrinkle and wither? Aging is ineluctable for animals and men. As death is for all beings, even including the angels and the gods. And this is so because dharma has programmed it, as it were, into its inner logic. Or, if you prefer, because the sovereign intelligence, always faithful to itself, has imposed the golden rule of reason: since essence is by definition eternal, then existence can only be transitory, mortal. Therefore everything that exists is subject to death: things, creatures, the gods themselves insofar as they are existents, and ultimately the universe, because it is the manifestation of existence (or existence itself). One day, all the parts of the Whole will be unmade and return to the state of undifferentiated matter (prakriti): existence will be reabsorbed into essence.

Pain, evil, is thus to exist, in other words to know that we are mortals and that all we love is perishable, doomed to destruction—even our chosen divinity, the one to whom our most fervent prayers are directed.[3]

The emotion experienced by the Hindu when he is made aware of this reality (and it happens at a very early age, since it is part of the most elementary religious instruction) is far stronger than any that can be inspired in us by the *Sic transit gloria mundi* of Christian preachers.

Christianity and Islam agree in viewing man as a creation (and therefore a "child of God") endowed with an immortal soul, capable of achieving his salvation during a single sojourn on this earth. That the world is a "vale of tears," that the Devil is forever striving to make men lose their souls, that men often succumb to temptation, all this is indisputable. But each individual, sure of the love God has for him, must hope to earn his place in heaven, provided that he himself participates in universal love and believes in the Revelation. In their totality, therefore, these religions are basically optimistic. Christians and Moslems live by the promise God has made to them: they will live with him in glory for eternity after the Last Judgment. Hinduism, on the contrary, offers transitory satisfactions only. True, the pious man can hope to earn a place in Vishnu's paradise (or Shiva's, or that of the Great Goddess, etc.), but he knows that his stay "above" will be no more than a moment in the cosmic duration—even though that moment may last for thousands of centuries—since that paradise, because it exists, will be reabsorbed, together with all the chosen inhabiting it, into the primal matter from which the next universe will be formed.

All is therefore subject to time, and that is why the *Veda* contains hymns dedicated to time as a sovereign power that has "engendered" the worlds and the gods (and thus, in practice, holds them in its power, as a father does his children):

> *He draws the chariot of the universe,*
> *Time with a thousand eyes*
> *that never grows old.*
> *It was he who brought existence,*
> *who engendered heaven and earth;*
> *through him the sun burns,*
> *in him are all existences.*
> *Lord of all that exists,*
> *he is the father of Prajapati;*[4]
> *in him live the Gandharvas, the Apsaras,*
> *on him the three worlds rest,*
> *and this earth, and the supreme dwelling-place.*[5]

Holding all beings and all things subject to its cruel law, time appears in the last resort as the intrinsic form of existence: to exist is to be inserted in duration, it is perpetually to transform the future into the past through an ungraspable present; whereas essence, because it transcends time, knows neither past nor future, but remains forever in the eternal present.

There is another source of suffering: existential plurality in contrast to essential unity. Brahman may be one, but beings and things are innumerable. The reader will recall the image of the cosmic wheel, its "thousand spokes," its circumference composed of the multiplicity of created things; gigantic, revolving endlessly around its center (for the length of one cosmic cycle), its fulcrum and motive force is the single axis of being, *tad*, "That," brahman. But multiplicity is division, dispersion; it is what separates us from one another. Situated in space and time, we suffer from inherent limitations, whereas essence is without limits; indeed, to speak of "localization" is to draw a boundary around the thing in question: it is here and not elsewhere, it occupies such and such a place in time and no other, etc. Where is its freedom in such a situation? Powerful king though he was, Ashoka could not escape from his age or his geographical domain: he lacked the power to transfer his kingdom to the moon or to take it back a thousand years in time.[6] He did bear the responsibility of his own actions in relation to dharma, but only within the narrow limits fixed by the necessity that caused him to be born into a specific family, in a specific place, on a specific date. To the Hindu, any freedom attributed to him is therefore illusory because it is merely relative: that is duhkham, suffering. Not that men do not enjoy a certain freedom to maneuver, but the pleasure they draw from that fact is adulterated because it is relative, transitory, so strictly determined. In the last resort, the joys offered to us during life are truly griefs, because they force us into awareness of their precariousness. This young girl, for example, smiling, desirable, advancing toward me: she is not coming to give me joy but to torture me, because I know that she did not exist yesterday and will no longer exist tomorrow. As I enfold her in my arms, I naively believe that communication is possible, that we are about to become one. But that is mere folly! She is separated from me by infinite distances, and the duality "she/I" is irremediable. We must be careful, though; this does not mean that Hinduism denies the reality of living beings: she exists and I exist too;

we are not shadows but individuals, whose existence is true because it is based on an essence (the soul; in Sanskrit, *atman*). In the same way, the happiness we feel at existing side by side has nothing illusory in it (otherwise it could not be the cause of suffering). The evil, the duhkham, I must repeat, is that she is "she" and I am "I," and that our shared pleasure is limited in time and space. As the Vedic scriptures say: "Where there is duality there cannot be happiness."

However, if it is true that man is analogous with the universe, then he must have a "center," a "fixed point" within himself, something equivalent to the hub of the cosmic wheel. And if this essential something is in fact concealed at the heart of the existential manifestation that is man, it is self-evident that it can only be That, tad, brahman, because the absolute is by definition one and indivisible. This, indeed, is precisely what all the traditional Hindu texts vie with one another in proclaiming: man is a microcosm exactly analogous to the macrocosm; and essence is present within him (as it is in every living being, moreover), "lodging," as it were, in the most inward part of him:

> *Tinier than the tiniest,*
> *vaster than the vastest,*
> *the Soul is inserted*
> *in the most secret part of the creature.*[7]

What is the *Upanishad* telling us here? First, that brahman, when it resides in the individual, takes the name of *atman;* and second, that this atman is responsible for that individual's existence, since the texts say that he is the "creature" of the atman. In other words, the translation of *atman* by "soul" should not lead the reader to suppose that the Hindu doctrine is similar to that of, say, Christianity. On the contrary, it is very different indeed. Where the religions derived from the Bible teach that souls are created by God as immortal (but not eternal) individuals, Hinduism teaches that the soul is nothing other than God (the Absolute) himself; it is therefore eternal and plays the same role within the microcosm as it does as brahman in the universe:

> *In the beginning, the soul*
> *which transcends all forms of existence*
> *moved upon the waters*
> *like a light breeze;*

in it the ego first made itself manifest,
the root of all things,
in which the three qualities came into balance. . . .
When it is affected
by the joys and misfortunes of existence,
it is called jiva, the individual soul.[8]

This second text has the advantage of bringing out clearly the divine role played by the atman: we see that the Absolute can equally well be called brahman or atman, God or soul, depending on which specific cosmic function is being attributed to it. Moreover, it clearly indicates that the appearance of self-consciousness (the ego) triggers the process of the soul's incarnation, and that once that soul has become involved in the process of existence it becomes a *jiva* ("one of the living"), an individual soul.

In strict logic, therefore, there ought to be only one atman identically present in all beings. This is the position adopted by certain schools, notably the *Vedanta* (particularly in the form handed down by Shankara). Yoga, on the other hand—faithful in this to another traditional current of thought, the Samkhya—prefers to teach that individual souls proceed from the universal soul and are multiple like the bodies in which they find incarnation. Just as dharma remains one, beyond the plurality of its existential manifestations, just as brahman remains the One-with-no-Second at the center of the multiple magic that constitutes the universe, so atman also is one in the midst of the numberless horde of its incarnations. It is at once true and false to say that souls are plural or that atman is singular: it is something that depends on the viewpoint being adopted. Metaphysically there is only one soul: essence, the Absolute, That, brahman, without name or form. But experience shows that living souls (*jiva-atman*) are in practice several. And yoga, because it is first and foremost practice, holds to the human viewpoint and accepts the experiential datum of the plurality of souls. Having done so, however, it strives with all its might—as we shall see—to "free" those souls by enabling them to return to their true nature, which is unity.

Whatever the differences on this point, it must be repeated that the atman is eternal and therefore indestructible, non-engendered, etc. As Krishna tells Arjuna in the *Bhagavad-Gita:*

The atman is not born and never dies;
it did not come into being and will not come into being;

> *non-engendered, eternal, permanent,*
> *it does not die when the body dies.*[9]

The implications of this passage are clear enough: if atman is eternal, where was it before the birth of the individual? Where will it go after his death? Krishna tells us in a later stanza:

> *Just as someone throws off used garments*
> *in order to put on new ones,*
> *so does the embodied soul throw off worn-out bodies*
> *in order to put on new ones.*[10]

This is the doctrine of transmigration (*samsara*, "the flow of change in all things") depicted very powerfully in one of the *Yoga Upanishads:*

> *It is happy, the child that sucks*
> *at its mother's breast;*
> *it is the same breast it*
> *fed from in a former life!*
> *The husband takes his pleasure*
> *in his wife's belly:*
> *it was in that same belly*
> *he was conceived in the past!*
> *He who was the father*
> *is today the son,*
> *and that son, when tomorrow comes,*
> *will be a father in his turn;*
> *thus, in the flow of samsara*
> *men are like the buckets*
> *around a water-wheel!*[11]

This passage brings us back to the symbolism of the cosmic wheel, envisaged here in motion: its circumference composed of the uninterrupted chain of deaths and rebirths undergone by the entire mass of living beings and irradiated by the vital energy pouring out from brahman (the hub of the wheel, the axis of the world).

During the lifetime of an entire cycle, often compared to a complete revolution of the cosmic wheel, beings and things, having emerged from undifferentiated matter, are made manifest in accordance with the laws of dharma (i.e. they are born, develop, waste away, and die), ceaselessly renewing themselves for an indefinite period (millions upon millions of times) until the final reabsorption of the three worlds into the primordial matter from which everything will begin again. In the *Bhagavad-Gita*, Krishna compares a cosmic cycle to one day from the point of view of brahman, followed by a night (a period during which matter, prakriti, remains as if slumbering before once more unfurling its magic beauties in the dawn of another day):

> *When day appears,*
> *existences are born from the unmanifested;*
> *then return into it in the evening,*
> *becoming the unmanifested again.*
> *Yes, these innumerable existences*
> *are ceaselessly born and reborn*
> *as long as the day lasts,*
> *and return, despite themselves, to the unmanifested*
> *in order to be reborn from it once again*
> *at the dawn of another day.*[12]

And as the world is organized in accordance with dharma, so its beings are too, as we have seen—into groups or species on the one hand, and as individuals on the other, by virtue of atman.

One *Yoga Upanishad*, for example, having recalled the presence of brahman at the center of the universe (and thus in the heart of each thing as the "best" of each) affirms that brahman likewise inhabits man as atman:

> *As the scent in the flower,*
> *butter in milk,*
> *oil in the sesame seed,*
> *gold in ore,*
> *That is in all things.*
> *Yes, the world's innumerable beings*
> *are shot through with the soul*
> *like pearls pierced by their thread.*
> *Yes, the soul runs through*
> *the worlds' numberless beings*
> *as the thread through pearls:*
> *like the oil in the sesame seed,*
> *scent in the flower,*
> *the soul is there in the body of man*
> *which it envelops and inhabits!*[13]

The final image is worth remarking on: atman is present in the individual's secret center, but from another point of view it can also be said to envelop him—in other words protect him, support him, give him his identity.

It now remains to see how samsara works. It might be thought that undifferentiated matter, when it begins to manifest itself anew at the dawn of a new cosmic day, allots a new role once and for all to each of the beings that emanates from it; or, if you prefer, one might envisage dharma as immutable, in the sense that each part of the great Whole, having once had its place determined in the general ordering of the cosmos, cannot change it during the next turn of the wheel. If that were so, the transmigration process would be purely mechanical: the human being would replace himself indefinitely, from the beginning of the cycle to its end, just as the species "ant" or "oak" would remain identical, not only as a species but even down to the individuals constituting the species. In other words, the spheres of existence would remain completely autonomous, juxtaposed, separate; the universe would be an archipelago.

Nothing could be more foreign to Indian ideology in all its forms, even including Buddhism in this case, than such a vision of the world: to the Indian mind nothing in the world of phenomena is static, constant, fixed; on the contrary, everything is in movement, everything is changing, undergoing transformation. Let there be no misunderstanding, however; dharma itself is permanent, immutable, because it is the Absolute; as the structure of things it remains always like itself, and this structure requires a fixed number of constituent elements; but the beings within this celestial machine move around, change places, make transitions from one function to another. If you will, the stock of living beings remains constant in mass, but each time an individual disappears, the place it occupied is immediately taken by another, which did not necessarily occupy the same role in its previous life. And the one that has just disappeared from the scene is sent back on stage to play a different part. To return to the example used earlier, the species "ant" and the species "oak" are both constituent elements in the general organization of the cosmos, and therefore immutable as such; but this particular ant, that particular oak, are living beings which, before returning in these forms, may have been a spider, a monkey, a brahmin, and after their deaths may become a scorpion, a Gandharva, or a pariah.

Here, of course, the notion of hierarchy, fundamental in all matters concerning the order of things, makes its reappearance. Since all beings occupy higher or lower positions (in relation to brahman/atman) on the cosmic pyramid, it will come as no surprise that the constant redistribution of roles required by the functioning of dharma is determined by each being's merits. Which means that any impression of anarchy created by a description of these continual reassignments is immediately corrected: dharma is present in everything, including the world's existential dynamic; for after all, is that dynamic not identical with life itself? Chance, it will be recalled, does not exist for the Hindu. Necessity and logical rigor are everywhere. Thus each being is responsible for its own destiny: each time it dies, the rebirth that follows must ineluctably be determined by a weighing of the actions performed during its life. If the scales tip on the side of good, then it is incarnated on a higher level; if toward evil, then it moves down to occupy a lower position, the distance downward being strictly proportionate to the degree of its demerits.

The *Manava-Dharma-Shastra* sets out an entire theory of the laws of transmigration,[14] based on the doctrine of the three cosmic qualities or gunas: sattva ("conformity with being," color: white), rajas ("passion," color: red), tamas ("shadows," color: black). According to the facts in each case, all our actions are ascribed to evil (tamas), to good (sattva), or to passion (rajas), which is an ambivalent category. The man who has done mostly evil in his life is reborn as an animal; the man who has done good rather than evil will find himself reborn as a genie, an angel, or even a god; and lastly, those who have allowed themselves to be ruled by their passions (according to the tradition, that is the case with the great majority of us) will be reborn once more as men or women. The *Manava-Dharma-Shastra* then goes on to list all the subdivisions that enable it to explain the existence of so many animal species, so many categories (castes) of man, so many celestial and divine "races." In addition, the boundaries between the three kinds of rebirth are shifting ones: barbarians (humans born outside India) and Indian outcastes are classified among the animals (and therefore ascribed to tamas), whereas certain denizens of the intermediate world, such as Gandharvas and Apsaras, share like high-caste Hindus in the dynamic of the rajas; the angels, the keepers of the stars, the mythical rishis, etc., are all "beings of the good," and therefore take their places in the domain of sattva with the gods proper.

Striving for complete systematization, the text even goes so far as to give a list of rebirths guaranteed to different types of sinners. Here are a few examples:

> *A brahmin who drinks alcohol*
> *will be reborn in the shape of an insect,*
> *a worm, a grasshopper; or he will return as a crow,*
> *or become a savage beast.*
> *Whoever steals perfumes becomes a muskrat,*
> *whoever steals vegetables a peacock;*
> *a man is reborn as a hedgehog after stealing cooked grain*
> *and as a porcupine after stealing grain uncooked.*[15]

Clearly the theory is not without its picturesque side. It is interesting to note too that the theory of transmigration does not exclude a belief in heavens and hells: before rebirth, the being can be kept for a time in one or other of these places. The *Manava-Dharma-Shastra* explains:

> *The souls of those who have acted ill*
> *take at their death another body*
> *as real as the one before*
> *and suffer the tortures of hell.*
> *When they have undergone in that other world*
> *the punishments that Yama was bound to inflict on them,*
> *the body dissolves, and its constituent parts*
> *reunite for another rebirth.*[16]

The idea here is that the body undergoing the suffering (or enjoying bliss in the case of those who have earned a stay in paradise) is a real one (since otherwise there could be no torture or pleasure), but different from the one assumed on earth, or in the atmosphere, or in heaven; which means that these heavens and hells, although situated like the three worlds within the sphere of existence, are different from them. Once again we recognize the Indians' analytic passion, their love of classification, and also their tendency to multiply categories, subcategories, etc., ad infinitum. More significant still is their determination to introduce everywhere into their structures an impeccable logic that totally excludes chance and reduces the operation of freedom.

Part 2

In Search of the Absolute

4. Knowledge

S amsara, it must be realized, is a source of suffering, an evil. It is part of the duhkham we have already seen embodied in the caste system and in the law of change that dooms the universe to ultimate disappearance, both in itself and in each of its parts. Not only is man mortal, but he must undergo this transition from life to death an indefinite number of times, not to speak of the sufferings inherent in his corporeal condition: disease, aging, grief.[1] To which must also be added the danger of sinking into hell and undergoing the most terrible of torments there before returning to the world for further rebirths. These various sources of suffering (or rather these various forms of evil-in-itself) are all allied, inasmuch as they are all a direct consequence of the simple fact of existing. In the essence/existence (or brahman/world) dialectic, existence is becoming and multiplicity, whereas essence is being and unity. At the beginning of each cosmic cycle, when the magic fabric (maya) of nature is unfurled—in other words when the world returns once more into existence—beings and things appear in such numbers that they cannot be counted, and the evolutive, dynamic characteristic of that nature, perpetually in the process of making and unmaking itself, is made manifest.

The Hindu scriptures put great emphasis on this vision of the manifest being unfurled at the very beginning of the world: the word itself used for "creation" is always a derivative of the verb root *srij*, "to emit" (we find: *srishti, visrishti, sarga,* etc., all having identical meanings); the idea is that of a "flowing out," a "diffusion," an "outpouring radiance," etc. Mythologically, Hinduism says that the supreme being experiences the need to multiply and to "manifest its glory" (in the words of the *Manava-Dharma-Shastra*), that "glory" being the light that dissolves the shadows in which chaos was wrapped. The beams emanating from the unique principle fertilize the primordial waters; a golden embryo appears floating upon them and the creating god, hypostasis of brahman, takes up residence within it. From that moment the process begins to accelerate: the demiurge separates heaven from earth[2] and produces beings and things by raising into place the constituent elements of matter (prakriti), the eternal substance symbolized by chaos (the Hindus say the "unmanifested") or by the primordial waters.

At other times it is the image of a cosmic man that is predominant, but the symbolism remains the same: in order to give the universe the form required by dharma, the creating deities offer up a sacrificial victim, the giant, the only being living beside the gods and a symbol of inert nature. Having been ritually dismembered,[3] he dies in order to give birth to the world, whose constituent parts are drawn from his substance: the sun is born from his right eye, the moon from his spirit, the wind from his breath, and so forth. Here again we find the themes of multiplicity (once unique, the cosmic man becomes innumerable), of becoming (the eye developing into the sun), and lastly of willed act, since this setting of the universe in place is the result of a ritual gesture. Many more examples could be given, other cosmogonic myths cited, giving expression to the Hindu feeling that existence is a plural agitation, perpetual change.

Hence, running through all the principal texts of traditional Hinduism, we find a yearning for unity and stability. In philosophic terms, the Hindu desires to pass from becoming to being; in religious terms, he hopes to be freed from multiplicity, in other words, from the necessity of unendingly being reborn. In short, he wants to leave the sphere of existence in order to rejoin essence, the principle that is absolute freedom because it is subject to no constraint, no limitation. This wish is called *mumuksha* (aspiration toward liberation, "desire to free oneself"), one of the fundamental dimensions of Hinduism and certainly one of the most original. It should be stressed that this aspiration toward liberation is not a desire to "go to heaven." Earning a place in paradise has nothing whatever to do with it, because paradise "exists" and is therefore subject to all the limitations inherent in existence (there are many paradises; they have specific locations; one only stays in them till a cycle ends; one sees God there but remains distinct from him, etc.) As it happens, many Hindus do "content themselves" with behaving as well as possible and displaying true piety in order to earn the reward of a stay in the paradise of their "chosen" deity. But they all know that this wish, though legitimate, is nothing in comparison with liberation (*moksha* or *mukti,* both derivatives, identical in meaning, from the root *muj,* "to liberate").

To understand exactly what this moksha is, we have to go back to the image of the individual's fundamental structure. Being analogous to the universe, he therefore possesses within himself a principle that cannot be different from the universal principle, because that principle is the Absolute and therefore, by definition, one and undivided. The atman within us is brahman, just as it may be said that brahman resides within the universe as its soul. Liberation will therefore be a function of the discovery (and of the "realization" as the sacred texts say) of the atman present in the inmost part of ourselves. In other words, in order for us to feel the desire to liberate our soul it is first necessary that we should become aware of possessing a soul and understand that it is not made for the fleshly condition at present imposed on it. In the first place, then, liberation is a matter of knowledge, and all Hindus agree in stressing this, since they all willingly concede that these two basic axioms (that we all possess a soul and that it was not made for existence) are not facts but rather articles of faith.

As one of the *Yoga Upanishads* says;

> *Living souls are prisoners*
> *of the joys and woes of existence;*
> *to liberate them from nature's magic*[4]
> *the knowledge of the brahman is necessary.*
> *It is hard to acquire, this knowledge,*
> *but it is the only boat*
> *to carry one over the river of samsara.*
> *A thousand are the paths that lead there,*
> *Yet it is one, in truth,*
> *knowledge, the supreme refuge!*[5]

However, the *Yogatattva Upanishad* would not be a true yoga text if it left things at that. Joining battle with those who teach that knowledge alone makes liberation possible, it goes on to tell us that the practice of yoga must also be added:

> *Without the practice of yoga*
> *How could knowledge*
> *Set the atman free?*

> *Inversely, how could the practice of yoga alone*
> *unbuttressed by knowledge,*
> *succeed in the task?*
> *The wise practitioner who desires liberation*
> *will direct his energies*
> *to both at once.*

We are reminded here that yoga is both theory and practice, albeit with theory predominating, since why should anyone commit himself to the hard path of apprenticeship in yoga without first knowing what he will gain by his struggle? The same *Upanishad* concludes its argument with this statement:

> *The source of unhappiness*
> *lies in ignorance;*
> *knowledge alone sets free.*

And this same doctrine, as I have said, is to be found in all the authoritative texts, not merely those in the field of yoga but those of all the orthodox Hindu schools. As an example, here is another passage from the *Bhagavad-Gita* (4.38):

> *There is nothing in the world*
> *that equals knowledge in purity;*
> *he who attains perfection*
> *through the practice of yoga*
> *discovers of his own accord, with time,*
> *the brahman present in his soul.*

We must not be misled, however, by that last line: it means that brahman (the text has *tad,* "That") is found in the secret recesses of the individual, and thus "in his atman," but since the Absolute can never be distinct from the Absolute, we are dealing once more with the equation atman = brahman, expressed here in symbolic terms.

Another of the *Yoga Upanishads* advances the notion that knowledge is "already there," that it is present in each one of us, even though the average man is not aware of it:

> *We know that milk*
> *is always the same color,*
> *even though the cows that give it*
> *have coats of different colors;*

just so knowledge is one,
even if the doctrines are diverse,
just like the color of the milk,
even though the cows are different.
And knowledge is hidden
in the depth of each individual
just as in milk
the butter we cannot see is hidden;
this is why the wise practitioner
must carry out a churning operation within himself,
employing his own mind without respite
as the churning agent.[6]

Whatever one's reaction to the image used here (internal butter making), the fundamental statement being made is a striking one: that knowledge is not something external to us to be received like a gift, nor a mental construction either, to be built up from scratch by logical reasoning, but that it is in reality a hidden treasure, something waiting in the very depths of ourselves to be discovered.

The images employed in the *Upanishad* just quoted—the color of milk (as proof of the unity of knowledge), the secret presence of the butter in the milk (constituting what is best in it)—are obviously allusions to the comparisons used by other texts to help us grasp the nature of atman/brahman. You will remember reading, a few pages back, that brahman is in all things "like the scent in the flower, butter in milk, oil in the sesame seed, gold in ore." The *Amritabindu Upanishad* was therefore clearly not selecting its image at random, and to say that knowledge is hidden within us like butter in milk is tantamount, in this context, to saying that knowledge is ultimately nothing other than the atman itself. So that the subject/object distinction is "transcended," in the Hegelian sense of the term. As the *Bhagavad-Gita* says (13.24.):

Through meditation
one sees the soul
in the soul, with the soul.

The idea being expressed by Krishna here is that when one practices meditation (that is, when one has reached the goal of yoga) one succeeds in seeing the atman (with "the heart's eye"), but that this vision can only occur "within the soul itself" and "by means of the atman" (*atmani . . . atmanam atmana*), because the sight of the Absolute is by definition unitary and must necessarily abolish all duality. There is therefore no longer any knower or any known but only knowing (knowledge), which is then coincident with the Absolute.

Moreover, the *Bhagavad-Gita*—in complete agreement here with the oldest *Upanishads* and the whole Indian metaphysical tradition— affirms that in fact the only knower is the atman itself. The reasoning is as follows: since beings are all sustained by atman/brahman, which irradiates them with its light and gives them life,[7] it is also that same Absolute which assumes responsibility, as it were, for the higher functions of existence (while remaining radically distinct from it). Thus when the individual, moved by the atman acting as "inner controller" (*antar-yamin*), strives toward true knowledge, the atman intervenes as knower. As the third book of the *Brihad Aranyaka Upanishad* says:

The atman, the immortal agent within yourself, is not seen but sees; is not heard but hears; is not perceived but perceives; is not known but knows. No, there is no other seer but the atman, no other hearer, or perceiver, or knower!

That [tad] is your atman, the immortal agent within yourself: all in you that is not It is doomed to suffering.

And the *Bhagavad-Gita* (13.1) makes use of a significant image when it says that the atman is the "knower of the field," or *kshetra-jna:*

> *This body that is yours,*
> *some compare to a field;*
> *and then he who knows it*
> *will be named Knower of the Field,*
> *according to the word of the ancient sages.*

And since Krishna is presented in the *Bhagavad-Gita* as being the soul of the world, he is also able to add (13.17):

> *Know then that in all the fields*
> *I am present as he who knows them;*
> *to know field and knower at the same time*
> *that is what I call knowledge.*

And needless to say, that knowledge leads on to the revelation of the atman's identity with brahman:

Light of lights,
we know that That is beyond the darkness;
being at once knowledge,
the object of knowledge,
and the path that leads to knowledge:
That resides at the heart of the universe.

The final line of that quotation is typical of the *Bhagavad-Gita's* intellectual method: in order to convey the total identity of the atman-knower with knowledge itself, with the method of knowing (yoga as "path"), and with brahman, the writer appends the statement that the latter—That—resides "at the heart" of the universe, exactly in the image of the atman present at the heart of man.

Now it remains to ask how this knowledge can be discovered. Being concealed, it remains inaccessible to ordinary mortals, and it is difficult to imagine how it could be reached by deductive reasoning. Is the reading of books (even the revealed scriptures), then meditating on their contents, sufficient to arouse this knowledge? If it really is transcendent, how can mere argumentation, even among theologians, ever rise above the level of existence (on which mental activity takes place) and attain to essence? As the *Yogatattva Upanishad* (1.7, 1.8) says:

No! this brahman by which all things,
from the sun up there to this simple pot,
are made manifest,
cannot be revealed by the scriptures.
That is manifested of itself;
That is beyond language
both human and divine;
That does not move, does not suffer;
That transcends all reality.

Of course, study of the scriptures can serve as a spur toward knowledge—and we shall see that yoga does not reject it a priori—but only on condition that we do not take it for an end in itself:

Certainly the yogi will be right
to digest the contents of the scriptures thoroughly
on condition that he later goes beyond this stage
and throws away all books,

> *as one throws away the chaff*
> *to find the grain!*[8]

There are many more passages of this kind that could be quoted, and it would even be possible to show that certain schools go so far as to say that study is more of an obstacle to the awakening of knowledge than a stimulus, since it incites men to vanity, to arrogance, and leads to a love of hair-splitting and irrelevant argument.

In practice, in order to trigger off the process that leads to realization of the unity of field and knower-of-the-field (to continue the image from the *Bhagavad-Gita*), the intervention of an external force, also derived from knowledge, is necessary. The reasoning is as follows: only the knower of the field can know itself; therefore, if the knowing power in a given individual is still asleep, a stimulus will be required from someone in whom the knower is awake. This person is given the name *guru,* meaning spiritual master.[9] Every man who has reached knowledge is capable of playing the role of master and taking disciples. But what is important is not to found a school but to possess skill in administering the initial jolt that will lead to the awakening of knowledge. It is significant in this respect that the very first prayer a young Hindu is taught, during his upanayana, is in fact called the "Incitress" or, in Sanskrit, *savitri.*[10] And this prayer, which every high-caste Hindu recites every day of his life from then on, is recognized, not unsurprisingly, as a goddess. Or to be more precise, as the manifestation "in prayer form" of the cosmic energy, *shakti,* that we shall be observing at work in the later stages of yoga.

What the guru provides is initiation. And, to be more precise, initiation into the third and highest stage of the religious life. Once more we encounter the hierarchic principle so characteristic of Hinduism. At the point when he reaches the age of reason (round about his tenth year), the boy of good family (i.e., one belonging to a jati) is obligatorily received into the first stage of religious life in an initiation ceremony that qualifies him to undertake his religious studies. He can be initiated into this first stage by his father, but usually it is a guru who admits him, and the boy then becomes the master's adoptive son (on the religious plane only). His studies should then continue, in theory, until the young man is in a position to set up a household of his own. When he makes this decision (though it is almost always the family that makes it for him), he informs his master, who then initiates him into the second stage, the one that ends his studies and raises him to parity of status with his father, his uncles, and any other adult males within the family who have similarly set up their own households in the past.

For the vast majority of Hindu males, everything ends there, since the number of those who become aware of a spiritual vocation in themselves is very small. Moreover, the scriptures are categorical on one point: if a man wishes to respect the law of dharma, he must always marry and beget at least one son before even thinking of setting out on the path of spiritual realization (either through learning or yoga). However, once a man has accomplished this essential duty of guaranteeing the continuity of his family line, he is free to embark upon that path if he so chooses. And if he does, then he must begin by seeking out a master capable of initiating him into the third stage, the guru who will stir up the knowledge that is still slumbering within him. This master may be the same guru who took charge of his earlier religious studies, though more often than not it will be some other master, known to the would-be disciple as a specialist in one particular sector of the tradition (in the words of the *Upanishad,* quoted earlier: "A thousand are the paths that lead there, yet it is one, in truth, knowledge.") And the scriptures are fond of saying that the quest for one's guru already constitutes an initiatory test whose duration will be proportionate to the seeker's merits.

At the end of this quest, when he has "recognized" his master, the disciple entrusts himself body and soul to the chosen guru, who eventually, after a period of novitiate, confers upon him the third and highest initiation that will open the "third eye,"[11] thus enabling his disciple to contemplate atman/brahman residing in the inmost part of himself. This moment is at once an end and a new beginning: it brings the years of apprenticeship to an end while simultaneously inaugurating the true task that lies ahead. In the yoga tradition, it is only after having received this final initiation that one may undertake the first exercises. In other words, initiation is neither an end in itself nor a guarantee of success. One may receive initiation and still not attain the supreme goal, which is a practical realization of the union of atman and brahman. The scriptures are quite clear on this point: in this domain also, many more are called than are chosen.

The reader will not have failed to notice that initiation is restricted to high-caste Hindus, that is, to those entitled to be called dvija (twice-born). Since they cannot receive upanayana, shudras, pariahs, and, even more so, non-Indians can never aspire to the third stage of an initiation from whose first and second stages they are by definition excluded. Furthermore, it is boys of the higher-caste families alone who are admitted, never girls. In other words, women are effectively excluded from the spiritual adventure too, and particularly from yoga. In practicing this discrimination, however, Hinduism is simply remaining faithful to the logic of its system. Upanayana is in practical terms the beginning of a religious apprenticeship with the purpose of instructing future heads of households in their daily ritual practices, all based on the obligation to offer up part of the food their households consume to the gods. The act of sacrifice can be performed only by a man,[12] whether it be in a private house or in a temple (where the priests are also exclusively men); girls, therefore, have no religious studies to undertake, and such studies are closed to them, just as the seminaries giving instruction to future Roman Catholic priests are still closed to women.

However, the wife does have a role to play in the household rituals, a secondary one admittedly but nevertheless ritually necessary. For this reason she receives a minor initiation from her husband on their marriage day, thus fitting her for the acolyte's role in the domestic liturgy that she will be called upon to play. Thus, one of the most important moments of the nuptial ceremony is the one at which the new bride walks around the ritual fire with her husband as her guide. At another point, as the groom pours an oblation into the fire for the first time—not just on his own behalf but also on that of his wife and the descendants she will give him—the young bride takes up a sitting position behind him and lays a hand on his shoulder: this is the procedure she will follow from now on, every day of her life, as mistress of the household, always taking her part in the ritual, but unobtrusively, in the role of a mute onlooker.

Minimal though this participation may be, it is nevertheless a fact. And one that certain traditions have taken as their authority for tolerating the presence of a yogi's wife beside him on his spiritual path. Only the yogi himself has actually undergone the major initiation, it is true, but his wife is nevertheless permitted to benefit from the spiritual radiance that her husband has acquired in the process. We know, for example, that Ramakrishna lived out his entire spiritual experience with his wife beside him: she waited upon him, prepared his meals, took care of his disciples' material needs, and so forth. And the Master stated categorically that this role, on the surface so humble, was imbuing her with such merit that her ultimate liberation was beyond doubt.[13] It must be stressed, however, that Ramakrishna's was a wholly exceptional case, and we must accept as a fact that the Indian tradition is fundamentally misogynist. It is perhaps not generally known that the word *yogini,* the feminine form of yogi, means "witch" or "female demon." Many passages from the scriptures could be quoted in which women who do dare to attempt the practice of yoga, or the acquisition of knowledge by some other means, are condemned to hell and then to the basest of rebirths.

Yet the discussion of Tantrism (see chapter 10 below) will show what a prestigious position this same tradition grants the eternal feminine.[14] It is likewise an easily observable fact that modern Hinduism is dominated by the worship accorded to the Great Goddess in all her forms. And those lucky enough to be welcomed into Indian homes will bear witness to the veneration that surrounds the mother and the respect inspired by young girls. But these are two orders of reality existing on different planes. On the level of daily life, as on that of religious devotions, the woman is sanctified by her role as mother (or future mother) and by the generosity of her gifts (the principal image being that of her freely offered milk, seen as a sort of sacrifice in which woman nourishes children with her own flesh); but at the same time the tradition insists on the fact that woman (and even more so the young girl) is the supreme temptation, turning men away from their spiritual quest. In this respect it is the erotic function that is given predominance: the all-powerfulness of *kama* (Love, son of Shiva) is indefatigably sung by the traditional authors.

But it is stressed—and this is another constant in the tradition—that the very thing that puts man in danger of falling should be used to help him rise in the spiritual hierarchy. Thus the provocative girl who maddens the senses and the mind is the very instrument that must be used if a man wishes to transcend existential temptation, progressing dialectically, in a manner of which we have already encountered some examples. This is the whole program of Tantrism, as we shall see later: advocacy of erotic practices to the end of spiritual realization. It should be borne in mind, however, that we are here at the very farthest limit of paradox; the more orthodox tradition remains more prudent (or, if you like, takes fewer risks) in advising the adept to avoid all contact with the feminine sex, and therefore to retire "to the wilderness" to receive initiation and advance along the path of spiritual realization.

5. *The Migratory Bird*

he aim of initiation is thus to give an aspirant the stimulus or spur, the savitri,[1] necessary to trigger off the process of awakening knowledge within him. What remains—the total realization of that knowledge—is for yoga to accomplish. However, before investigating the eight stages of classical yoga, perhaps it would be best to acquire some idea of what exactly the content of this knowledge is, since it will then be easier to understand why the long path that leads to liberation (moksha) is necessary, and why it should follow the particular itinerary it does. As you might expect, given Hinduism's passion for analysis and its predilection for ternary divisions, the tradition breaks the acquisition of knowledge down into three phases. First, there is the revelation of the atman's captive condition, then that of the causes of this alienation, and finally that of the ways that can lead to the imprisoned soul's liberation. The various texts do differ slightly, of course, in their accounts of the stages to be gone through before knowledge in all its plenitude may be obtained, especially with regard to the exact number of subdivisions involved. We find the *Vedanta Siddhanta Darshana,*[2] for example, giving a seven-runged ladder:

> *Seven are the levels of knowledge,*
> *the great prophets taught:*
> *the purity of the desire to know*
> *comes first; second, reflection;*
> *third, acuity of mind;*
> *to perceive what reality is*
> *and lose the taste for worldly things*
> *are the fourth and fifth levels;*
> *on the sixth, the object itself fades away:*
> *there is nothing left but the fourth state*
> *into which one enters*
> *on the seventh plane.*

As we shall discover later, this ladder displays a remarkable coincidence with the successive stages of yoga, even though the vocabulary here is that of the *Vedanta* (for instance, *turiya,* the fourth and final stage in this scheme, corresponds with what the *Yoga-Sutras* call the stage of *kaivalya,* "isolation," while the disappearance of the subject/object distinction corresponds to *dhyana,* "migration," etc.).

To return to the simple ternary division, which is by far the most natural and the most frequently employed by the texts, it is significant for us that the first stage should be the revelation of the soul in its captive condition. And as so often, the *Upanishads* here employ a specific symbolism to drive home their meaning—in this case the image of a migratory bird entangled in a birdcatcher's net. Indeed, if one thinks how the atman is condemned to pass on from body to body, for the duration of a whole cosmic cycle (except in the very rare instances of liberation), then this comparison with a migratory bird—*hamsa,* is a very natural one. (The actual species denoted by *hamsa* is not quite certain. It probably means the wild goose, but European translators have fought shy of that equivalence because of the goose's aura of peasant stupidity in Western popular tradition. It is often rendered by "swan" or "flamingo," though "crane" would probably be better.)

The *Hamsa Upanishad* (1.5) explains:

> *At our birth it enters into us*
> *the migratory bird! Like the fire*
> *invisibly present in the wood,*
> *like the oil hidden in the sesame seed,*
> *it dwells in the deepest depth of us:*
> *to know that is to free oneself from death.*

At each reincarnation it is as though a dove, alighting for an instant on the ground, finds itself once more imprisoned in the hunters' nets. So yoga, following the image through, will be one of the methods employed to cut through the net:

> *As a migratory bird,*
> *imprisoned by a net,*
> *flies up toward heaven*
> *after the threads of the snare holding it captive*
> *have been cut,*

so the soul of the adept,
liberated from the bonds of desire
by the knife of yoga,
escapes forever
from the prison of samsara.[3]

Before analyzing this passage more closely it would be as well to add that the atman-hamsa image is strengthened, in the yoga context, by a secondary symbolism derived from a direct phonetic-symbolic link between the act of breathing and the name of the migratory bird. When we breathe in, the texts ask, does not the air as it enters make the sound *ham?* And when we breathe out, does not the air hiss as it leaves, making the sound *sa?* So that we are all of us, however unwittingly, forever repeating *hamsa! hamsa!* And the yogi, having become aware of this phenomenon and its esoteric meaning, transmutes the two sounds into a prayer, which he then dedicates to his atman so that it will help him to reach the fullness of knowledge and so conquer death:

The air goes in making ham!
It goes out making sa!
So the living being lives life
repeating endlessly
the mantra of the bird!
One needs only to become aware of this
to be free from all sin.[4]

The use of the *mantra* in Hinduism needs little explanation. A mantra is a magic formula of supreme efficacity when manipulated by "those who know." Here, the Sanskrit name of the migratory bird constitutes the entire mantra, and its perpetual repetition relates to the *japa* (repetition) technique with which we shall be dealing later on.

It should also be added that the same two syllables in reverse order (with a slight phonetic change required by the rules of Sanskrit grammar) mean something quite different: *so'ham, so'ham* ("I am It, I am It") we also all proclaim as we breathe, and "It," needless to say, is hamsa, the atman. Again, moreover, consciousness (a real, effective, experienced consciousness) of the secret meaning of the two syllables *so'ham* has a liberating power. By repetition of this new mantra (esoterically identical with the first), one obtains liberation because one is "realizing" the identity of the self with the inner controlling force (antar-yamin)—yet one more name of atman/brahman. Combined, the two mantras are an encapsulation of the entire doctrine: "I am it, that migratory bird!" In other words: "My true self is the atman there in the deepest heart of myself!"

We still need to know, however, how the soul has come to be imprisoned in this way, what exactly these toils are in which it is tangled, and why they are there. In short, to find out the cause (probably single) of transmigration. What we have learned about dharma in previous chapters should enable us to guess in which direction to search: since the gradual breakdown of the cosmic order manifests itself at human level in an increasing disharmony in social behavior (increase in the number of castes, progressive barbarization of mankind, etc.), it may be supposed that individuals, inasmuch as they are all analogous to the universe (and thus to dharma in all its forms), are also participants in this disharmony, so that their attitudes ought to provide a translation of the situation into concrete terms. Now social behavior and individual attitudes exist primarily as actions; therefore it is at the level of actions that the process of the atman's alienation occurs. And all the texts do in fact concur in saying that it is action (*karman*) that is responsible for the soul's captivity.

There is a theological difficulty here that we must not try to gloss over: is the bad (contrary to dharma) action an effect of the growing cosmic disorder or its cause? Since the tradition speaks of an ineluctable degradation of dharma, expressed in the theory of the four cosmic ages, it seems natural to infer from this that our debased human behavior is merely one of the many forms of *adharma* (evil as the "contrary of dharma"). The individual behaves wrongly because he lives in the Kali-Yuga (the worst age of all), where everything conspires to "lead him into temptation." How could he possibly observe all the rules of dharma when the "tongue of the gods" (Sanskrit) has ceased to be a living language and is no longer understood by more than a mere handful of learned men who have had to work hard for years in order to master it? Ultimately, it is hard to see how there can be any talk of individual responsibility when we know that each one of us is rigorously determined by the conditions of his birth (he hasn't chosen to be born in this or that jati) and, perhaps even more rigorously, by his social environment.

Unanimously, however, the scriptures counter such fatalism by say-

ing that the freedom of the individual remains total, whatever the
conditions under which it is exercised, and that the value of the merits
and demerits acquired in a life is obviously relative to the location (in
time and space) of the particular activity being considered. It is a
point we saw made earlier: the duties of a pariah are not those of a
brahmin; indeed, it is upon the distinction between those duties that
the metaphysical justification of the caste system rests (by analogy with
the distinction between species: the dharma of a wolf is different from
that of a lamb). Hence Krishna tells Arjuna:

> *It is better to accomplish*
> *one's natural duty, even imperfectly,*
> *than to follow to perfection*
> *the laws of another group;*
> *to perform the duty appropriate to one's status*
> *cannot be a sin.*[5]

If, then, the impossible were to happen, if everyone were to perform
perfectly the duties required by his *sva-dharma* (dharma proper to
him), then sin would not exist and the world would be in perfect
balance. But the world and the individual both belong to the sphere of
existence and consequently assume all its qualities: dynamic change,
activity, multiplicity. Subjected to the necessity of living, beings cannot
refrain from acting, since life is an indefinite chain of actions that individually and as whole are both the causes and the effects of all those
that have preceded them in time and all those that will follow them.
Krishna explains again:

> *No one in fact can cease to act,*
> *not even for an instant:*
> *all are constrained to action,*
> *even against their own will,*
> *by their natural predispositions.*[6]

We cannot escape this law, even though we may imagine we are
capable of remaining at rest. Just as we cannot stop time, so we cannot
break the dynamic chain of cause and effect.

Furthermore, since life (dharma) is, in itself, growth, aging, death,
rebirth, the actions performed cannot *not* contribute to the propagation
of life. For a being, the mere fact of existing entails, as we have seen,

its integration into the "common flow" (samsara) of transmigration. And this fact transposed onto the dialectical level of being and acting may be expressed as a law: action (karman) determines life, which is to say gives the living being (jiva) its place in the hierarchy of creatures. So the doctrine of karman is no longer merely a corollary of the ideology of dharma but appears as its true metaphysical basis:

> *Whether one acts in thought,*
> *in words, or in deed,*
> *the act accomplished*
> *will bear fruit, good or bad,*
> *and determine the future life*
> *better, equal, or lower.*[7]

To act in accordance with the dharma proper to one's birth is to guarantee onself the prospect of being reborn on at least the same level (and possibly on a higher one); to go against the universal norm entails certain down-grading (with the possibility of a sojourn in hell beforehand). That is the ineluctable law, the living expression of the existential condition, which, in this sense, recognizes each individual's freedom to act well or ill, together with all the consequences of that freedom. The vast majority of Hindus, as we saw earlier, accept this situation and do their best to act in accordance with their caste dharma throughout their lives. But what of those who become possessed by the "love of unity" and try to escape from the "common flow," even though acceptance of it holds out the promise of delight in paradise to those who act in holy accord with it?

   In good logic, since it is action that determines becoming, not to act should suffice to interrupt that becoming. However, to remain in the realm of logic, there is a possible objection to this. Any interruption of samsara in an individual who succeeded, by some miracle, in ceasing to act would not mean the abolition of transmigration but simply a halt in it, which is quite different; this non-acting being would then find itself frozen in an indefinite existential present. I should add at once, however, that this is a philosophical position held by no more than a very few Hindu thinkers, usually drawn from the ranks of practitioners of bhakti (devotion). These thinkers do in fact depict liberation quite often as a cohabitation of the freed soul with its Lord, and according to this point of view the two subjects involved (God and the individual atman) both exist but do not act: they live out of mutual and indefinite contemplation that is the very definition of their cosmic status. But views of this kind, so close to those expressed by Christian theologians, are not typical of Hinduism; they fall into the realm of universal religious feeling, and on that account stand outside the problematics of yoga, which is what alone concerns us here. We shall therefore return to the basic doctrine of the great traditional scriptural texts, which teach, it will be remembered, that all felicity—however high—remains relative (and therefore metaphysically bad) as long as it is no more than a specific form of existence. Strictly speaking, the devout being enjoying the grace of cohabiting with Vishnu in paradise is experiencing no more than an illusory happiness within the realm of the universal maya.

Moreover it is impossible in logic to conceive of an act that would bear no fruit, in other words an act that would be pure consequence, without effect. To Hindu thinking, the single, independent act does not ultimately exist: action is seen rather as a melodic line that coincides with life itself. This being so, it is not possible to imagine a form of existence exempt from causality. Liberation cannot be anything other than an emergence from the sphere of existence, a return to essence, a transition into transcendence. Of course, because it is "essential," brahman does not act in any way, and the atman—merely a name given to brahman for convenience when referring to its presence in the human person—likewise remains impassive, non-acting, etc. So we are apparently once more facing the necessity of proposing the same solution: in order to obtain liberation, man would need, "like brahman/atman," to not act. And yet, does not dharma teach us that brahman is "the principle" (i.e., in strict logic, the cause) of all things? Is it not written that "That" is the initial spur that gave Vishvakarman the desire and strength to build the cosmic house we all inhabit? Does Krishna not tell Arjuna that the atman is the knower? And, lastly, do not the scriptures celebrate "That," tad, brahman, under the trinitary name sach-chid-ananda (being-consciousness-joy)? So it cannot be the act-in-itself that is bad, since it is quite evident that knowing, inciting, etc., are acts. Presumably the badness lies in a particular type of act, a type for which all we beings-in-the-world, from the humblest of creatures up to the great gods themselves, have particular fondness.

Existential acts can, in effect, be assigned a value quotient. The theory is, as we have seen, that "one becomes good by good action, bad by bad action." Becoming is therefore certainly linked to the value of the action in relation to dharma. Moreover, although it is true that each act is the consequence of all those before it, the principle of causality does not function in accordance with some elementary mechanical model in which every action is the immediate effect of the one situated just prior to it in time. The system is much more complex; it presupposes that the totality of its past actions is weighing on the living being at the moment when he is about to perform an act, so that the resulting act remains free (since the faculty of choice remains), while also being determined by the weight of karman anterior to it (i.e., by the totality of past acts that have now become causes of the future act), which manifests itself as a predisposition to act.

It is such a predisposition that manifested itself as the original incitation, the intial stimulus, from which our world emerged. To that predisposition, that stimulus, the texts usually give the name *kama* (desire, love), and say, for example, that in the beginning the Demiurge "desired to multiply himself"; and the cosmogonic hymn in the *Rig-Veda* (10.129.4) also celebrates kama as "that which developed first" at the beginning of the world.

On more than one occasion this results in the cosmogonies taking an erotic turn; it is explained that the initial kama manifested itself in the form of a drop of divine sperm falling into the primordial waters. Thus impregnated, the waters produced a golden embryo (also called *brahmanda*, "egg fertilized by Brahma") from which the universe emerged. Love is thus undoubtedly the sole cause, the principle "beyond the gods":

> *Love was born first;*
> *the gods cannot reach it,*
> *or the spirits, or men. . . .*
> *Far as heaven and earth extend,*
> *far as the waters go,*
> *high as the fire burns,*
> *you are greater, love!*
> *The wind cannot reach you,*
> *nor the fire, nor the sun, nor the moon:*
> *you are greater than them all, love!*[8]

It is the first manifestation of life, which in the last analysis is identified with it (so that the phrase "God is love" is accepted by traditional

Hinduism, which recognizes the supreme existent as kama "first-born, first hypostasis of brahman-essence").

By analogy, it can be said that desire moves in the heart of man as a primary (and permanent) stimulus emanating from the atman. In a sense, therefore, it can be said that the golden embryo (thus assimilated into the atman-knower) is present in the most inward part of us, where it is constantly developing through the agency of our acts. And it is our responsibility to give it good and beautiful form. From this point of view the love that supports the world is quite clearly a beneficent force:

> *The worlds would dissolve into nothing*
> *if I ceased to act,*

Krishna tells Arjuna (*Bhagavad-Gita*, 3.24). It should be remembered that Hinduism is to the vast majority of its faithful a *karma-marga*, a "way of good works," dharma in action. Nor should we forget that the word *karman* denotes primarily the ritual act, religion as something "acted" (i.e., "lived," and therefore "oriented" in some specific direction). The whole of the *Veda* is a continual paean of praise to sacrifice as karman, the act par excellence. Moreover it is said of the head of a high-caste household that his whole life is lived in terms of one golden rule: *svarga-kamo yajate*, "desirous of reaching heaven, he performs the acts of worship."

Krishna also says:

> *Nourished by sacrifice, the gods*
> *will grant you the graces requested.*[9]

This means he is both guaranteeing the devout Hindu that he will assuredly win his way to heaven, the object of his desire, and also revealing (since Krishna is the supreme god instructing man in the truth) that the cosmogonic power is the sacrificial act (karman) born of desire (kama).

For, as the *Rig-Veda* also says (10.90.8.):

> *From the universal sacrifice*
> *the gods received the Butter,*
> *from which they drew forth the beings*
> *that people the air, the forest, the villages.*

As you might imagine, the bhakti (devotion) doctrines make much use of the scriptural passages that express views of this kind. And we also find the *Mimamsa*—one of the great *darshanas* (traditional systems for explaining the world)—constructing an entire metaphysics based on the act of creation in order to justify action in the world. This is the darshana of the most rigorously orthodox brahmins, assiduous in their duty of offering up every day, night and morning, the sacrifice of *agnihotra*[10] which "supports the world" (it is said that the universe will vanish when the last brahmin has celebrated the last agnihotra).

In opposition to this view, however, we find that the masters preaching liberation look upon this compliance with karman (in its highest form: sacrifice) as the worst of all dangers:

> *Some seek their path*
> *in the practice of rites*
> *as the Veda teaches:*
> *they fall, through ignorance,*
> *into the trap of ritualism.*[11]

For these masters (and naturally the champions of yoga are among the most virulent of these critics of the scriptures), the *Veda,* holy though it is, is valid solely on the plane of life as existence: it contains the divine instruction that enables men to attain to the highest forms of that existence, but not how to go beyond (except to certain sections of the *Veda*—notably the *Upanishads*—in which the identity of brahman and atman is expounded). It is in this sense that the scriptures should be construed as a mask of ignorance concealing the face of truth. And this is an image that we find, for instance, in the *Bhagavad-Gita* (3.39), when Krishna explains to Arjuna that knowledge (i.e., the atman/truth as knower) is rendered blind by desire (kama):

> *Knowledge is masked*
> *by the veil of evil*
> *that has taken the form of desire,*
> *permanent enemy of the wise man.*

So now we know the formula: it is not a question of ceasing to act, since that is impossible within the sphere of existence, but of acting while at the same time eliminating as far as possible all desire.

> *He who performs the prescribed act*
> *without concerning himself with the fruit it bears,*
> *he is the ascetic, the true yogi,*

Krishna tells Arjuna (6.1). And what the divine guru is telling his disciple here is that it is not necessary to renounce the practice of the rites in order to achieve liberation, but that one must strive to continue acting in accordance with dharma while "forgetting" the primary motivation of one's actions, which in this case is "the desire to win a place in heaven."

If one succeeds, then one's atman finds itself released from existential contingencies and ceases to suffer: for it, good fortune and bad, renown and scorn are equally without interest. And having attained equanimity, in the literal sense of the word, one will attach no more importance "to a golden coin than to a pebble," as the *Bhagavad-Gita* (6.8) puts it.

The program at least is now perfectly explicit: if the atman finds itself caught in the toils of transmigration, it is because it inhabits the body of a living being, and because life is action; if the individual acts, it is because life is desire and because it is not possible to cease to live (i.e., to leave the sphere of existence) without ceasing to desire. If one could succeed in doing so, then the atman would be suddenly released:

> *Free of all desire,*
> *the adept becomes immortal;*
> *released from temptations,*
> *having cut the thread*
> *that held him in the world,*
> *he is now released forever*
> *from the bonds of samsara.*[12]

I must repeat once more that the adept in question here does not stop acting, he only stops desiring; motivated action is both consequence and cause, but disinterested actions (in the strongest sense of "disinterested"—being free from all attachment) cannot bear fruit; the individual in this stage of spirtual development "does nothing" because the deeds he performs have become purely mechanical, anodine, without interest for him:

> *When he has renounced*
> *attachment to the fruits of all works,*
> *even-minded, independent,*
> *he does nothing*
> *although held in the whirlpool of doing.*[13]

This is the condition of the *jivan-mukta* (the "liberated-alive"), which will be described later, in the discussion of what happens to the yogi as he attains the last rung on the ladder of yoga. For the moment, let us turn again to Krishna:

> *Desire has set up its seat*
> *in our senses, our mind, our intelligence;*
> *making use of them, it conceals knowledge*
> *and deceives the individual.*
> *We think our senses can help us,*
> *and our mind, and our intelligence,*
> *but desire is stronger than they.*
> *Knowing that desire conquers even the intelligence,*
> *it is by the atman that one must strengthen*
> *the atman and strike at desire,*
> *the elusive enemy!*[14]

6. From Yogas to Yoga

We have just seen that various methods are proposed for releasing the migratory bird trapped in the toils of samsara. We have heard about knowledge, about bhakti, about disinterested action, etc. And it seems likely that still other methods may exist that have not yet cropped up in the course of our investigations. It is now time, I think, to present a systematic account of these various paths available to the individual setting out on "the quest for the Absolute." And the first thing to be said is that all of them are referred to as *margas* or as *yogas*. The first word means "path" or "road," so that *jnana-marga* is "the path of learning," a method that uses intellectually acquired knowledge as its preferred means of obtaining liberation. As for the word *yoga,* that of course is the one of prime interest to us here.

First, then, what does the word as such actually mean? It is derived from the root *yuj* (to harness), and its primary meaning is "the action of harnessing." Thus in the very oldest of the Vedic hymns we read of the horses that are harnessed to the chariots of gods such as Indra (personification of warlike strength) or Surya (god of the sun). Such contexts have the advantage of emphasizing the values of violence and constraint that have remained fundamental to its meaning through the word's history. In fact, it is worth stressing that despite the existence of the Latin noun *jugum* (English "yoke") from the same Indo-European sources, *yoga* has never meant "yoke" in Sanskrit: the tranquil operation of yoking oxen evokes a peaceful, pleasant way of life that has nothing in common with yoga.[1] For the yoke is something used by vaishyas and shudras, whereas the harnessing of horses is a task for kshatriyas. This last point becomes even clearer when we know that the chariots (*ratha*) we read about in the *Veda* are always military vehicles, battle chariots. Krishna, after all, instructs Arjuna in yoga while standing in a battle chariot of which he is the driver, and their dialogue (the *Bhagavad-Gita*) takes place just before a great battle is engaged.

When we add to the simple action of harnessing horses the notion of the skill or art involved in that process, then we are moving toward the secondary meaning of *yoga:* "magic recipe" or "method." For example, when the *Yogatattva Upanishad* (1.74) tells us that "by means of yoga" one can "with the help of a little mud mixed with urine transmute brass into gold," the word *yoga* is given the meaning of "magic recipe." This aspect of the discipline is so important in the view of its masters that one of the four books of the *Yoga-Sutras* is entirely given over to it.

Nevertheless, "method" is the meaning most often intended in the scriptural texts. It may be used with reference to any of the disciplines, and particularly when it is a matter of giving "technical instructions" for the correct execution of the Brahmanic rites. Derivatives such as *niyoga* and *viniyoga* signify nothing more than "prescription" or "user's instructions," as it were. For example, one will read that a particular mantra[2] has its prescribed use (niyoga) in such and such a liturgical context. At other times the same terms are used to denote explanations of how a specific substance is to be used, or of what particular posture to assume during a ceremony, etc. Then in speaking of a plan, a project, or the process of preparation (especially mental preparation), another derivative is used: *prayoga,* the meaning of which later shifted toward the actual work being executed, the project in the process of realization; hence the meaning "good execution" or "staging" in the case of a play. So much for the semantic field covered by yoga the noun. We shall find that its implications as a *name* become apparent of their own accord as we progress.

As we know, Hindu tradition is almost exclusively preoccupied with establishing the laws of dharma on the one hand—so that the right order of things shall be preserved as long as possible—and, on the other, with educating the few worthy of it in the various paths that will enable them to achieve liberation. This latter aspect of the tradition finds expression in numerous texts that may be termed "metaphysical" (although "metareligious" would really be better, since what is involved is an esoteric theology rather than a general philosophy). These texts are divided among six great "systems" called *darshanas* (viewpoints), because although they all claim to be expositions of one and the same doctrine, they all approach it from a different angle.[3] One such text, the *Nyaya,* bases its argument on deductive principles, hence its name "logic"; another concentrates on detailed and pains-taking exegesis of the Vedic scriptures and is therefore known as *Mimamsa* (hermeneutics); and so on. The interesting thing from our point of view is that yoga appears in the list of six darshanas under "Method." Which is as much as to say that in the eyes of the Brahmanic tradition it is the "technical" darshana par excellence, the one that signposts the path in a concrete way to those "in search of the Abso-lute." All the basic texts of the *Yoga-darshana,* indeed, are devoted to the description of spiritual exercises whose purpose is the attainment of a particular state that will make possible the transition from existence to essence—the transition, it will be remembered, that actually consti-tutes liberation.

Upon reading these texts, however, we find that within the general yoga framework a variety of methods is being put forward, and not just one as might have been expected. In the *Shiva-Samhita* (5.14), for example, we read:

> *Four are the methods:*
> *they are named:* mantra-yoga,
> hatha-yoga, laya-yoga;
> *the fourth is* raja-yoga:
> *through it one transcends all duality.*

As for the *Bhagavad-Gita,* that balances *karma-yoga* against *jnana-yoga* and develops what might be called the "program" of *bhakti-yoga!* These are only a few of the names that recur most often, and it would not be difficult to extend the list: *tantra-yoga, Shiva-yoga,* etc. And the *Bhagavad-Gita,* as though to make it clear that the list remains perpetu-ally open, gives each of the eighteen chapters a title that includes the word *yoga:* thus the first is the "yoga of confusion" (*vishada-yoga*); the fifth "the yoga of renunciation" (*samnyasa-yoga*); the eleventh "the yoga of the vision of cosmic form" (*vishvarupa-darshana-yoga*), and so on.

This is a way of teaching that any procedure whatever can be made use of in the quest for the Absolute on condition that it is given the value of yoga or, in other words, harmonized with the basic principles of yoga as such. From this viewpoint, even the confusion Arjuna experiences just before engaging in combat is worthy of being raised to the rank of a spiritual exercise, inasmuch as the hero, under the direction of his divine guru, becomes capable of transcending it, of changing it—by means of a genuinely alchemical transmutation—into a necessary (and therefore salutary) stage on the path of yoga.

There is therefore no reason to insist at length on the multiplicity of "yogas." A few words will suffice on those most frequently mentioned in modern works (above all since they were described by Vivekananda in the late nineteenth century).

¶Karma-yoga, as its name indicates, is a spiritual method that proposes to keep the adept in the world (and therefore to lead him to accept the necessity of acting in accordance with dharma) while also teaching him how to avoid the fruits of karman (action). If the master succeeds in extinguishing all appetite, all desire from his disciple's consciousness, then action on the part of that disciple is freed from the law of causality; no longer having any effect, it no longer constrains the individual to be reborn after his death. In practice, karma-yoga is usually combined with bhakti-yoga (yoga of devotion), since it is accepted that the practice of disinterested action is more or less impossible to realize without a special grace from the Lord:

> *He who performs his duties fully*
> *while taking refuge in me,*
> *attains, by the effect of my grace,*
> *the eternal, immutable world.*[4]

Krishna's teaching here is categorical: it is the grace of the Lord (*prasada*), not personal effort, that makes possible the transition into the essential sphere. Personal effort, however, is necessary as a precondition of receiving the grace; seen like this, yoga consists in fulfilling one's caste duties while constantly fixing one's thoughts not on what one is doing but upon the Lord: that is the entire program of bhakti-yoga. One must take care to remember, however, that this type of yoga is not simply advocating the ordinary observance of one's religious duties: such everyday devotional practice falls into the realm of "ordinary" devotion and leads the faithful Hindu to a place in paradise, whereas bhakti-yoga—precisely insofar as it is a form of yoga—is directed at the achievement of liberation.

The same can be said of jnana-yoga, which makes use of intellectually acquired knowledge to obtain the release of the captive soul. At first glance, the method here seems to consist solely in studying the scriptures, meditating upon them, and delving ever deeper and deeper into their meaning—in short, in theological study. But that can be no more than a preliminary stage, and one in which must not dally for too long (remember that all the texts quoted earlier go so far as to say that books are an obstacle on the path to liberation); the real aim of this study is to awaken the knower/atman within oneself in order to receive from it a clear vision of the road to be taken. Here again, the *Bhagavad-Gita* and most of the other texts advocate a combination of jnana-yoga and devotion; for is the atman-knower not the "inner controller" (antar-yamin) or, in other words, the Lord himself? Is the individual not "his own creature"?

> He who with the help of devotion
> succeeds in knowing My true nature,
> thus knowing Me at last in truth,
> enters with his prayer into Me.[5]

The last line of that stanza is an opportune reminder that the aim of jnana-yoga is indeed to achieve liberation: the man who succeeds in attaining supreme knowledge (that of the atman-Lord's "true nature," *tattva*) goes on to "enter into the Lord," to dissolve into him, thus realizing "in truth" the unity of knower and known.

All these different sorts of yoga are no more, however, than variants (and in many respects aberrant ones) of classical yoga, the only one treated unanimously in the tradition as the valid reference, and described for this reason, when the need arises to give it a specific name, as raja-yoga, "royal yoga," or rajadhiraja-yoga, "yoga of the King of Kings." This last name (which refers to one of the titles of Shiva) has the advantage of calling attention to the part played in the formation of classical yoga's rules by the Shivaite tradition: Shiva is venerated in them time after time as *Maha-yogin,* "the Great Yogi," the patron of all those wishing to take the path of yoga. It is with this total yoga that we shall be dealing in the following chapters, precisely because it is the supreme form of the discipline, the immutable structure into which all the specific methods favored by any particular yoga school must eventually be inserted. And in fact, many of the names give to these ancillary yogas are actually no more than references to the various stages or rungs of raja-yoga. Hatha-yoga, the "yoga of strength," for instance, which puts all its emphasis on physical exercises, is no more than a somewhat extended development of classical yoga's third stage (the one concerned with postures), just as tantra-yoga, so described because some *tantras* describe it at great length, offers a detailed analysis of what exactly is taking place during deep meditation (dhyana, classical yoga's seventh stage). Sometimes, in fact, the reference is merely to a subdivision within a stage, as with mantra-yoga, the "yoga of magic formulas" which deals with the magical efficacy of the specific words or phrases employed to help concentrate the mind, etc.

In short, it might be said that nouns such as bhakti-yoga, karma-yoga, jnana-yoga, and so on, function as adjectives. The first is a form of raja-yoga in which the adept is aided in his progress by devout worship of his *ishta-devata* (m., chosen deity—the god or goddess to whom the Hindus give preference in their ritual devotions); the second concentrates on the method that consists in practicing raja-yoga while remaining in the sphere of worldly life; the third justifies a taste for intellectual inquiry by integrating it into the various stages of classical yoga, and so on. As occasion arises, I shall indicate during the remainder of this book what specific "coloration" these various types of yoga may give to the fundamental method, but without concealing the fact that masters of integral yoga are sometimes forced to warn their disciples against the danger of self-indulgence lurking in the practice of these "secondary methods." Jnana-yoga, for example, as we have already seen, entails the risk of immersing the adept so deeply in the delights of theological dispute as to make him forget that such exercises are no more than a tool (whose purpose is to detach the mind from worldly things), not an end in themselves. Similarly, any attempt to continue acting in the world while at the same time claiming to practice yoga must entail the risk of engendering a secret love of action, a love that may eventually blossom into the desire to act. And that would mean the loss of all the efforts already made to achieve one's liberation.

I shall therefore follow the tradition in asserting that there is only one yoga. And I shall attempt to present it systematically, in its integrity —a method that will lead me to employ not only the *Yoga-Sutras* and the commentaries on them, but also the *Upanishads,* the *Tantras,* the *Bhagavad-Gita,* and the various compilations accepted as having a traditional authority, such as the *Shiva-Samhita,* the *Hatha-Yoga-Pradipika,* the *Gheranda-Samhita,* etc. But as an introduction to this synthetic view it may be useful if I give an account of the way in which all these texts conceive of the "human composite," the microcosm in which existence and essence cohabit, man the object-subject within which all the cosmic powers are permanently at work.

The soul/body dichotomy, so dear to Western theologians, is not unknown, as we have seen, to the Brahmanic tradition, which makes an unequivocal distinction between all that partakes of existence and That (tad, brahman, atman), which is essence itself, the Absolute. On the macrocosmic level, this is the dialectic of purusha (spirit, essence, Absolute) and prakriti (matter, existence, nature). And man, by analogy, is at once flesh and spirit, soul and body; his atman, like a migratory bird, is imprisoned in man's carnal condition. However, this simple dichotomy does not wholly satisfy the Indian mind, which has a natural tendency to conceive of things in terms of a ternary rather than a binary structure. So, like certain Western traditions, it prefers to posit the structure *spiritus/anima/corpus* as being closer to reality than the sequence *anima/corpus,* which lacks, in its eyes, the necessary link element permitting a comprehension of how existential phenomena (for example actions and their consequences) can come to have an influence on impassive essence. In the *Katha-Upanishad* we read:

> *The body is like a chariot*
> *of which the soul is the owner;*
> *the intelligence is its driver,*
> *the mind plays the part of the reins;*
> *as for the horses, those are the senses;*
> *the world is their arena.*[6]

In that passage we find yet again the metaphor of the chariot, one that has always been a favored tool in the teachings of the yoga masters.

The terms used in our last quotation require some explanation. First, we must remember that in Ancient India the battle chariot always belonged to the aristocrat wealthy enough to finance its construction, and that it was this owner who fought in it (usually as an archer). Also, this light but rather inadequately harnessed vehicle (the horse collar had not yet been invented) was very difficult to handle, which conferred great prestige on skilled charioteers. The guild of *sutas* (chariot drivers) constituted a high-ranking jati belonging to the varna of the kshatriyas. And Vishnu incarnated himself as the driver of Arjuna's chariot. In this form—as Krishna, that is—he will not actually fight, but he will nevertheless do everything within his power to see that his master emerges from the battle victorious. The *Upani-shad* quoted above is therefore quite right in making the atman the owner of the chariot, a supreme function corresponding well with that of the inner controller (antar-yamin), while the intelligence/driver (*buddhi*) plays the part of liaison agent between the soul and the chariot, whose motion it controls by means of the reins and horses. Here again the hierarchical gradation typical of Indian thought is clearly visible: the body (chariot), a material mass passive in itself, is moved by the organs of perception and action (*indriya*), which the *Upanishad* identifies with the horses drawing the chariot; these organs are governed by the brain (*manas*), whose activity is in its turn inspired, spurred into action, by the buddhi, the driver responsible for the fate of the vehicle, the holder of the reins.

If we try to schematize this structure, we are led to represent it as in figure 1.

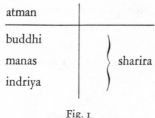

Fig. 1
The human composite

This makes it quite clear that the atman (because it is essence, the Absolute) is radically different from the totality formed by buddhi (intelligence), manas (thought), and indriya (organs of perception and action) which together form the body (*sharira*) in the full sense of the term, since they all belong, individually and together, to the sphere of existence. And this is why Krishna could explain, in the passage quoted at the end of the previous chapter, that "desire" (kama) is superior to the senses (indriya), to the mind (manas), and to intelligence (buddhi).[7] The same schema, applied on the macro-cosmic level, can be used to express the purusha/prakriti (spirit-essence/matter-existence) dichotomy. Thus in our second scheme we find the body's three constituent elements corresponding to the three

divine "species": the senses are the *devatas* (minor deities), the manas
is Indra (king of the divine cohorts), the buddhi is Ishvara (the Demiurge, the Universal Maker). But, as we know, all the gods "exist"
and therefore partake of prakriti, whereas atman/brahman is purusha
itself (see figure 2).

atman	brahman	purusha
buddhi	ishvara	⎫
manas	indra	⎬ prakriti
indriya	devata	⎭

Fig. 2
Constituent elements of the human composite

You will have noticed the central position allotted to the manas, in
which it corresponds to nothing less than "the king of the gods." This
is because it is the source of activity and actually controls the horses,
whereas the buddhi's role is primarily inspirational (on the human psychological level) or creative (on the cosmic level).

Hierarchically, however, the buddhi remains the summit of the
corporeal complex, a position that brings it as near as possible—while
still remaining within the realm of prakriti—to the atman. And the
relations between soul and intelligence are sometimes difficult to define.
We have already seen, for example, that the atman when "incarnated"
(the jiva-atman or "living soul") is the knower. And it is also described as the "inner controller" (antar-yamin). Yet these are the
very roles that one would like to see played by intelligence. The
Bhagavad-Gita, on the other hand, depicts Krishna as a charioteer (i.e.,
fulfilling the role of the buddhi) revealing the truth to his passenger
Arjuna, who is the embodiment of the atman! This is an astonishing
paradox that can be justified only within the context of bhakti (devotion): Krishna has voluntarily come down to earth in order to save
dharma;[8] but this entails his assuming the highest possible position
within the world of existence, that of Ishvara (the Lord), which is to
say, within man as microcosm, that of the buddhi. The scriptures usually say that the Demiurge is a hypostasis of brahman in the existential
sphere. And the buddhi, on the human level, might be called the corporeal manifestation of the atman. In this sense, the buddhi translates

into human language something of the transcendental knowledge that the atman in itself is.

Hence the idea that the inspirations radiated by the buddhi are normally good but remain veiled (and therefore hard to decipher) by the mask of ignorance created by desire.[9] If the individual succeeds in listening with the requisite attention, he will hear the voice of the intelligence, which is no other than that of Ishvara (God). This is why the Hindu tradition locates the buddhi in the heart, where the atman itself also resides. Thus the knower, the inner controller, diffuses its invisible light, and the buddhi, even when sullied by the impurities of desire, always reflects something at least of that radiance. One of the aims of yoga is thus to lead the adept toward an inner vision of his own heart. And if the adept manages to free himself from desire, then his buddhi will suddenly reflect not just a gleam but the full radiance of his atman (as we know, liberation is sometimes depicted as a sudden illumination of the whole being). Nevertheless, the buddhi in its role as reflection of the atman provides no more than a discreet assistance. It is always available, if one wishes to address oneself to it, but normally it contents itself with simply maintaining the fragile human composite in a state of equilibrium. The buddhi leaves all the work of life to the manas, which alone plays a truly active role, just as Ishvara is the father, the judge, the guardian of dharma, while the actual administration of the world is in the hands of Indra, king of creation.

Yoga is therefore concerned in the first place with the control of mental activity, as the first sutra categorically states: *yogash chittavritti-nirodhah,*[10] "yoga is the cessation of mental activity." The word *chitta* denotes everything that is "thought, conceived, perceived, conscious," and *vritti* evokes the notion of "whirlwinds" (the noun derives from the root *vrit,* to turn). Thus the idea being conveyed is that the life of the mind consists of an uninterrupted succession of thoughts all linked one to another, rather like the separate frames of a movie film that produce an impression of unbroken movement when projected at a specific speed; or like the waters of a river whose very swirling melds them into one continuous flow; or again (and this is probably the true symbol buried in the word *vritti*) like the circle of fire traced in the air by the myriad flames that Shiva juggles with when he is depicted as Nata-raja (Lord of the Dance). The important thing to grasp, at all events, is that in the eyes of the Hindu tradition the manas can never be at rest. Belonging as it does to the world of existence, it is a permanent dynamism, multiplying and diversifying its activity to infinity.

It goes without saying that this agitation is in the highest degree "distracting" and diverts the individual from his quest for the Absolute. The din it sets up within us is such that we are unable to hear the voice of the intelligence, with the result that we allow ourselves to be swept along in its eddying flood, not just without resistance but even with pleasure, with active compliance on our part, just as the spectator at a movie or the listener at a concert, transported into a world different from his own, will forget for a while his preoccupations of the moment. And yet, incoherent and disordered as this agitation may at first appear, it is so on the surface only. For India, as we have seen, does not believe in the random, and the Hindu tradition explains this inevitable mental whirlpool with its theory of *vasanas*. The word *vasana* means "impregnation, latency," as when one speaks, for instance, of a cloth retaining the scent of a flower momentarily laid upon it. We speak in rather the same way of "retaining the impression"—whether pleasant or unpleasant—of a meeting with someone or a view. However, it is as well to avoid using "impression" as a translation of vasana because it evokes the mechanism of memory. Although that mechanism does seem at first glance very close to what is intended by vasana, the two things are in fact different, for a vasana is always the result of an action performed by the subject, never of an "external aggression" passively undergone (and can the Hindu manas ever behave passively?).

By acting in a given way at a given moment, I bend the future fate of this being I call "me," however slightly, in a direction I am not yet aware of, because at the moment I perform that action my being is impregnated with a certain "odor" (subtle, imperceptible, inconceivable by the ordinary mind) of the cosmic value of the forces involved in that action. In the Christian tradition, something of the sort was probably being recalled when, as a result of actions performed, a person was said to be "in the odor of sanctity." And it should be stressed that it is the entire personality that is affected by each vasana. Or, if you prefer, it is constructed, vasana upon vasana, as a house is built brick by brick. And for Brahmanism, of course, such a process could not possibly be broken off at an individual's death or begin absolutely afresh at birth; vasanas are accumulating from the very beginning of each cycle for each being, and continue to increase in number, as one continues to perform acts, on until the end of the cosmic cycle. Thus we are all "impregnated" with all the karman we have amassed during all our previous lives, all perpetually preparing our future destinies by our unending activity (since the actions in question are mental as well as physical, and one is being impregnated even by one's dreams).

Needless to say, since nature (prakriti) is always recreated out of the same basic material, the vasanas are not creations ex nihilo (the Indian mind finds the notion repugnant), but rather the effects of perpetual transformations. Since each of our actions as it occurs is motivated by our previous karman, it is as though every particular action we perform burns up the particular vasanas immediately responsible for the impulses creating that moment. But, since the act performed "bears fruit," new vasanas appear that are in fact modifications of their predecessors. And so we are back with the image of the mental whirlpool, the perpetual vortex. The task yoga therefore sets itself is to destroy vasanas without producing new ones. A difficult program to carry through, since the acts the average man performs each day burn up only a very small fraction of the vasanas he carries within him (which is why he will have to be reborn again and again). If the yogi does succeed in reducing his activity to a minimum, the mass of stored-up impregnations that abruptly manifests itself is enormous. It is as though a dam had burst and let out a whole lake all at once, so that we find descriptions in all the texts of the terrible mental phantasmagoria that explodes at the moment when the adept attains meditative nonactivity—descriptions in which one immediately recognizes the universal symbolism of the "temptations in the wilderness." But if the individual holds firm, then this explosion will prove to have been the crowning-piece of a mental firework display; the vasanas will at last have been burned off, and their disappearance will enable the yogi to take a great step toward liberation.

As for the body proper, apparently deprived of all prestige by its hierarchical position as the very lowest of the constituents of human nature, the use that yoga puts it to is well known. And with good reason, since corporeal experience (the simple conscious sensation of having a body) is a preliminary precondition to embarking on the path of yoga. The first step the adept takes will therefore to be "realize" (i.e., to know intuitively) this miraculous tool that he can put to such a variety

of uses. Attentive to the organic quality of life, conscious of the pro-
found unity of the individual I am, I shall be led by my commitment
to the path of yoga to meditate in the first place upon my body (we
know, for example, that yoga advocates concentrating the attention on
specific areas of the human body: the tip of the nose, the navel, etc.).
My body is in fact a reflection of my inner life, the mute witness of its
struggles: it shows me to myself. I cannot detach myself from it; for
better or worse we are indissolubly bound together. Nothing, in fact,
could be more foreign to the Hindu tradition, and in particular to the
form it takes in the *Yoga-darshana,* than any attempt to sever the inner
life from corporeal life: life is one, and such distinctions are at best
no more than convenient pedagogic devices. Which is why spiritual
action (the means of liberation) must occur on all levels at once and
involve the body just as much as the manas and the buddhi. Moreover,
the body is itself a paradox: it contains within it the inexhaustible
wealth we seek; yet it is endowed with hands that reach out toward the
outside, eyes that look outward, legs that lead it away from itself: it is
like a lord laying waste a great fortune of which he is the trustee. Here
again yoga will make use of the very existence of the body and its particular characteristics to constrain it to assist the individual in achieving
liberation. Those arms and legs that stretch out toward the external
world will be bent back, twisted together, pressed against the body as
though to protect the inner wealth (the atman); those eyes avid to contemplate the magic glamor of phenomena will be closed; and so forth.
In this way the paradox will be annihilated; the body will rediscover its
true function, which in the words of the Vedic hymns is to be "the
coffer in which is locked away that infinitely precious treasure the
atman."[11]

Part 3

The Royal Art

7. *Taming the Body*

To the aspirant who presents himself and begs to be granted the grace of acceptance as a disciple, the guru replies first with a warning: yoga is not for the weak; it requires physical vigor and strength of character. Not just firmness of purpose, upright intention, and wholeness of body,[1] but also readiness to submit to violence and to exercise it upon oneself. For the path upon which the disciple is to embark is that of a *sadhana*. This keyword in the Indian tradition refers to the act "of subjugating, of conquering, of overcoming" and is widely used in such contexts. From there it is but a short step to the meaning of magical action and, more specifically, of incantation. But it is clearly the meaning "spiritual realization" or, better still, "means to be used" in bringing about such a realization that concerns us here. In many respects Hinduism regards yoga as the supreme *sadhana* (*sadhaka* is another word for yogi, with the meaning of "he who has achieved the goal of yoga"), because it entails the use of methods of subjugation directed at the individual in his totality—body, thought organ, intelligence—whereas most of the other sadhanas (including magic) require the use of no more than a fraction of the forces present in man. Moreover, yoga is a one-way path; having reached its end, the adept is transformed from top to bottom by the operation of a subtle alchemy that achieves irreversible transmutations. Once transformed into gold, lead can never become lead again (and the basic yoga texts insist on the fact that the jivan-mukta[2] will never again return to the world of samsara, whatever he may do). And it is precisely because yoga is the perfect sadhana that it is reserved for the small elite of those who possess the inner resources necessary to sustain such an effort. The first task of the guru must therefore be to decide whether or not an aspirant does possess those resources, since this is a domain in which self-delusion is not easily avoided.

That the help of a master is obligatory during one's apprenticeship in yoga is a self-evident fact that no Hindu would dream of questioning. The tradition is handed on exclusively from guru to disciple, and no one could ever conceivably invent anything in the domain of truth, simply because truth is one and eternal. Having been revealed in its perfect entirety at the beginning of the cosmic cycle, this truth is to be found residing in an ever decreasing number of individuals as that cycle continues and dharma becomes increasingly degraded; and its depositaries, having themselves received it through initiation, must hand it on in the same way to those they judge worthy of receiving it. Moreover, when the sadhana toward which a man feels himself drawn is as technical as yoga, then it is obvious that he cannot help but become the pupil of someone who, simply because he is the repository of its technical details, must naturally stand in the office of a teacher.

In India, the group formed by master and disciples constitutes what is usually called an *ashram*.[3] It is better to retain this term untranslated, since it does not correspond to anything we are familiar with in the West. More often than not, the master is in practice a wandering ascetic to whom those desirous of gaining some spiritual advantage from his company are naturally drawn by his inner radiance. Sometimes the ascetic in question (he is called *sadhu,* "saint") does not in fact teach at all. There are many, for example, who have made vows of total silence; but the mere fact of seeing a sadhu, of observing his behavior, of meditating in his presence, is held to be of spiritual benefit. However, the "saints" we are concerned with here are those who do teach, and it is around them that the true ashrams are formed. In practice, these sadhus are very quick to pick out from among the merely curious or pious who come to them those individuals capable of becoming disciples, and at a certain point they give them a sign (since it would be improper for the future disciple to make the first move) and give them a number of rules to be observed during their novitiate. Later on, when the master judges that the aspirant has proved himself sufficiently, he grants him initiation and adopts him as his disciple. Not until then does the teaching proper begin.

The wanderings of the sadhus (and therefore of their ashram) is broken off by force of circumstance during the monsoon, and it is during this period of the year (June to October) that the ashram functions as a school. Many masters, of course, remain in one spot all the time; having halted there one year when the rains came, they have never moved on. Huts have been built by the faithful, and the community has settled in this theoretically temporary encampment. And in some cases, especially today, certain masters even agree to the construction of large, overtly permanent buildings and allow the ashram to become a structured institution.[4] It must be stressed, however, that this phenomenon is a departure from the orthodox norm (in the eyes of Hindu tradition, needless to say) and is visibly modeled on Western institutions. The true ashram is totally "open"; one goes there when one wishes, lives there as one wishes, and leaves it when one feels like it, and the master does not involve himself in any kind of administration. In fact there is nothing to administer, since the individuals who live for a while beside a master make it their own business, individually, to find their own food and shelter for the night. Only the true disciples (those who have been initiated and are therefore considered the master's spiritual sons) have any duties with regard to the guru: finding him food, seeing to his needs, protecting him from troublesome visitors. Normally, the question of money ought never to arise, since everything necessary for life should come from unsolicited gifts. Local villagers and curious visitors bring the necessary daily fare, while in the larger ashrams the disciples go on a begging round every day, or ask for alms from the inhabitants of the neighboring town. Master and disciples must never engage in any activity involving remuneration, and the wisdom acquired by initiation can never be sold.

Both master and disciples (initiates) are what are called "renouncers" (*samnyasin*), men who have solemnly declared their determination to withdraw from the world and who, from that moment on, find themselves cut off from everything that constitutes the ordinary fabric of life in the world—external activities, family bonds, social advantages. This renunciation (*samnyasa*), it need scarcely be said, stands in direct conflict with dharma. To live as the head of a family, to take over control of the family after the death of one's father, to observe scrupulously all the social rules of one's jati and varna—these are absolute obligations, and to fail in them is to sink back after death to the lowest rung of the ladder of beings. In such an order of things, there is no place allotted to those who voluntarily withdraw from the exercise of their natural function in the world.

To this the masters reply that by living in the world a man can indeed earn his upward progress through the hierarchy of beings from rebirth to rebirth, and that he may be granted the grace of remaining until the end of a cycle in the paradise of a god. The gurus, on the other hand, are seeking the definitive release of their atmans and, having understood that transmigration is perpetuated by the effects of all actions performed, have renounced action altogether. But the risk is immense, since to fail in this quest for the Absolute is to lose everything after a wretched life spent in discomfort and solitude. Indeed, it may be the very precariousness of the "renouncers' " earthly existence (and consequently of their extremely small numbers in relation to the vast population of the subcontinent as a whole) that has led Hindu society to tolerate their existence. Inversely, that very tolerance has acted as a "safety valve": it probably explains why such a restrictive society has never exploded. Paradoxically, it is samnyasa (renunciation) that has saved (and is still saving) the caste system.

India thus accepts that certain of her sons contest her social order, to the point of rejecting it; and she does so magnanimously, in that the renouncer is sure of never dying of hunger—it is highly improbable that he will ever be refused alms. Moreover, village communities traditionally construct a shelter near their settlement (but outside it) where pilgrims and sadhus may take temporary shelter. Such institutions (daily alms, building of a *dharmashala*) form part of the body of pious works that guarantee the giver great merits, and in this way the community takes the samnyasins under its wing.

At the same time, however, the community takes great care to keep itself apart from these individuals who have renounced it: the sadhu is impurity in the absolute, because he no longer observes the rules of caste. He is truly one of the walking dead, since he renounced his civil status at the moment when he left the world (Hindu law stipulates that his wife acquires the status of a widow, and that his heirs inherit, at the instant the samnyasin pronounces his vows, etc.). The *Manava-Dharma-Shastra* specifically lays down that the renouncer must have no possessions other than a staff and a bowl for alms (6.41), that he must never enter the house of a dvija,[5] and that he must never beg for his food until evening, when the villagers have all eaten their meal (6.56). Most sadhus wander about, wretched and half-starved, existing on little more than a daily bowl of rice or a little fruit, powerless to better their lot since they must beg only once a day, with the result that the vast majority of them succumb to malnutrition and disease in a very short time.

I have felt it necessary to emphasize the real conditions of daily life experienced by most renouncers in order to make it clear that samnyasa, the preliminary stage of yoga, is no light matter. The scriptural texts, because they are solely concerned with those who succeed, tend to sing the praises of renunciation in such a way that the unwary reader could well acquire a very false impression of what it means in concrete terms.[6] On the other hand, although Hindus avoid all social contact with the samnyasins because they are ritually impure, it is also true that they are always ready to listen to them and favorably predisposed toward whatever they have to say. Any individual who stoically accepts such conditions of existence must be doing so for motives powerful enough to merit the interest of all. Consequently the visit of a sadhu is always an event in any village, and all the more so in that his appearance will be picturesque and his behavior unusual.

In India, where an individual's caste (or, at least, his varna) is always clearly apparent at a glance, simply from his clothes or the way he wears his hair, etc., the sadhu is immediately recognizable by the piece of orange-colored cloth (in his case it is the color that is specific) that he knots around his loins (or wears after the fashion of a toga— but in every case the garment consists of a simple length of material, neither shaped nor sewn); above all, the renouncer must never cut a single hair on his body from the moment he pronounces his vow: long hair, beard, and mustache are the visible outward signs of his status. Usually the hair is plaited into fine braids and knotted on the top of the head (Shiva, in his role as Maha-yogi, uses the crescent moon to keep his knot in place). Many sadhus wear necklaces, especially rosaries of large beads made from various kinds of wood, according to the deity they have chosen as their preferred object of meditation; the staff sometimes becomes a trident if the sadhu is a Shivaite; the body bears ritual markings made with ashes or colored dust. It is easy to understand how these holy beggars excite public curiousity!

Those who practice bhakti-yoga (and there are a great many of them) are often musicians and singers. Accompanying themselves on a tambourine, castanets, tiny cymbals, or some stringed instrument, they sing devotional hymns that the villagers never tire of hearing, and these sadhus at least are guaranteed as much food as they can eat. The practitioners of jnana-yoga tend to preach sermons, engage in theological debates with the local pandit,[7] give advice to the troubled and occasionally allow themselves to be persuaded into performing a little magic, astrology, or alchemy. If they have strong personalities, if what they have to say or sing has value, they inevitably find people following

them in their journeyings for a while and it is not long before some of
these followers become their disciples, by mutual consent. At this point
the sadhu becomes a guru, and an ashram forms around him.

What has just been said on the subject of samnyasa and transmission
by initiation should make it clear that the master/disciple (guru/
shishya) relationship has little connection with the educational system
we are used to in the West. To find anything equivalent in our culture
we would have to go back to our Middle Ages, to the days when
students paid their professors themselves and lived with them in small
communities. The future disciple, once accepted as a novice by his
master, must declare his intention of renouncing the world to his family
and share out his worldly goods among them. He then entrusts his
wife and children to his brother (or father) and, in a specific ritual
ceremony, takes leave of the domestic hearth upon which he has
hitherto poured his daily libation of milk.[8] From this moment on, the
guru will be the only link connecting him in any way with the external
world:

> The guru is his father, he is his mother,
> he is his god too, beyond doubt.
> The disciple will serve him
> in act, in word, in thought.[9]

Which is to say that the disciple's life, during the entire period he
remains a member of the ashram, must be that of a devout worshiper
in constant veneration of his chosen deity. The same text makes this
clear when instructing him how to approach his guru:

> Advancing toward his master
> he will walk three times around him;
> and, touching his feet with his hand,
> he will greet him lying flat on his belly.[10]

A totally prone position is the sign of absolute submission, and Hindu
tradition reserves it for the worship of the major gods.

It will readily be gathered therefore, given such a situation, that
casting doubt on one's guru's utterances is strictly inconceivable.
Moreover:

> Salutary alone is knowledge
> received from the lips of the guru;

for all other is barren,
without value, dangerous.[11]

The *Shiva-Samhita* even goes so far as to specify that in the ideal pantheon constituted for the disciple by the guru and the tutelary gods of study, "the guru is on the right" (i.e., in the place of honor) while Ganesha,[12] Vishvakarman the Maker of the cosmos, and the goddess Ambika are all on the left of the altar, in the place traditionally allotted to secondary deities (*Shiva-Samhita,* 3.22.).

Patanjali's *Yoga-Sutras,* which form the foundation of the yoga-darshana, divide the path leading to liberation into eight stages. Hence the name "yoga in eight parts" (*ashtanga-yoga*) sometimes applied to the discipline we are studying. These eight stages or degrees are:

1. *yama,* restraint;
2. *niyama,* spiritual discipline;
3. *asana,* posture;
4. *pranayama,* breath control;
5. *pratyahara,* withdrawal of the senses;
6. *dharana,* mental concentration;
7. *dhyana,* deep meditation;
8. *samadhi,* higher consciousness.

Before examining the various stages in detail it is worth remarking that they can be grouped together in twos. In a moment, for example, we shall see that yama and niyama are learned and practiced simultaneously. In the same way there is no discontinuity between dhyana and samadhi, the latter being merely a deepening of the former, and so forth. This simplification into four "great stages" enables us to discern an equivalent structure to the one we met earlier underlying the "human composite." There we found three elements (indriya, manas, buddhi) contrasted with a fourth (atman), which transcends them absolutely. And here it is clear that stages 1 to 6 are concerned with psychocorporeal disciplines that we might term ordinary, since they employ means common to other fields (moral values, physical exercises, techniques of concentration), whereas the last two, as we shall see later, are specific to yoga: dhyana is a form of transcendental meditation similar—hardly surprisingly—to the Japanese zen,[13] while samadhi, the realization of the supreme identity (atman/brahman) is an emergence from the existential. The resulting scheme (figure 3) exactly reproduces the division of figure 1, derived from the structure of the human composite. This is an interesting additional indication of the coherence of Hindu thought, as well as good evidence of how closely all the elements of yoga are integrated.

IV	8. samadhi 7. dhyana	spirit
---	---	---
III	6. dharana 5. pratyahara	
II	4. pranayama 3. asana	body
I	2. niyama 1. yama	

Fig. 3
The human composite and the eight stages

The first two stages, yama and niyama, together constitute the first period of yoga apprenticeship—the novitiate. This means that the aspirant has now been recognized by the master as possessing the necessary dispositions for yoga. But before conferring initiation on him—that is, before adopting him definitively as a disciple, with all the reciprocal duties implied in the relationship—the guru puts him to the test of inviting him to show proof of his aptitude. It must be clearly understood—for this is an important point—that the novice has already solemnly renounced the world and is now living in the ashram. If, therefore, he does not prove successful in his novitiate, he will be forced to set off once more on his wanderings in search of another master, for he cannot go back home again. An apprenticeship in yoga is not for the average man: it is a matter to be settled solely between inhabitants of the same world, the sadhus, or samnyasins, whichever you prefer to call them.

The verb root *yam* from which both yama and niyama derive (and which recurs in the name of the next stage: pranayama), signifies "to tame"; it is used particularly to denote the act of breaking in wild horses and compelling them, against their will, to accept being harnessed to the chariot they are to draw. Needless to say, there is nothing random about the choice of these two words—rather than any of the many other possible ones—to denote the first two stages of yoga: an animal tamer is precisely what the aspirant must become. He must tame his instincts, his worldly inclinations, his desires, and channel the forces they embody toward a new goal. Patanjali specifies that the "restraints," or yamas, are five in number: (1) not to harm living beings, (2) not to lie, (3) not to steal, (4) to abstain from sexual relations, (5) to eschew covetousness. One's first impression of this list of ethical commandments is that they are hardly of great originality. The adept might point out, for example, that he has never been a thief, and that since he has renounced the world he no longer has any opportunity for covetousness.

It would then be the guru's duty to explain the five restraints to him one by one, in order to show that they must be practiced on a heroic scale, since their primary objective is to lead the future disciple to an awareness of the vasanas (psychic impregnations) he carries within him. These impregnations will erupt with a violence proportionate to the sincerity of the novice's renunciation of the world, and play the role of temptresses. His sexual appetites in particular will manifest themselves with great acuteness during sleep, and as long as they are present one cannot speak of true chastity, since India attributes no less reality to acts one performs in dreams than to those one performs when awake. Vyasa, the first commentator of the *Yoga-Sutras*, also explains what the second yama (truthfulness) should be:

Yamas and niyamas all have their root in ahimsa [not harming living beings]; their aim is to perfect this love that we ought to have for all creatures. . . . Now to speak truth is to bring our actions into harmony with the words we speak. One speaks only in order to communicate to others the knowledge one has acquired by looking, listening, deducting. To say that one has used the power of speech for the good of others is possible only if the knowledge communicated has not been deceptive, confused, or barren. However, even if it were not willfully deceptive, confused, or barren, and were still prejudicial to another for some other reason, then it would not be the virtue of truthfulness: it would only be one more sin. Consequently one must reflect with care before uttering a word and speak only out of love for others. (Yogasutra-bhashya 2.30.)

Thus "not to lie any more" does not merely mean to strive to speak the

truth, but also to take care that no word uttered is in danger of bringing harm to another. The yamas, then, are not just negative but positive too, and the positive value may even be said to be preponderant,
as Vyasa explains. (We should also note here the emphasis placed on
the virtue of ahimsa, which has dominated Hindu thought from the
Upanishads to Gandhi).

The niyamas too are five in number and are clearly practiced simultaneously with the yamas. Here is the list given in the *Yoga-Sutras*
(2.32): (1) to be clean, (2) to retain equanimity in all circumstances,
(3) to practice asceticism, (4) to study, (5) to be devout. Here again
the master must explain that what is required goes beyond the words
used. The cleanliness required, for example, must manifest itself at
every level of the human composite; not only should the novice keep
his body scrupulously clean, but he is urged to "wash" his mind thoroughly too by systematically rejecting all impure thoughts, etc. The
ideal aim is to wash away one's vasanas just as one washes dirt from
the body, though at such an early stage the novice's efforts in this domain can be no more than preparatory; the unconscious impregnations
do not evaporate definitively until samadhi is achieved.

The other niyamas may be the subject of argument and vary according to the teachings of different gurus. However, all agree that
number 3, *tapas* or "ascesis," consists, as Vyasa says in his commentary
(*Yoga-Sutras* 2.32.), in "going beyond the contraries that characterize
existence, such as hunger and thirst, hot and cold, the desire to stand
and the desire to sit," and so forth.

Here we encounter a mode of thought typical of the Indian tradition: life in the world is conceived of as a permanent conflict between opposing desires impossible of simultaneous satisfaction (in
India one does not drink with meals; one must therefore choose between appeasing one's hunger or one's thirst). Tapas (ascetic virtue)
thus consists in mastering one's desires in order to transcend this dialectic, which is seen as a manifestation of sarvam duhkham ("all is
suffering").

Arguments do arise, on the other hand, on the subject of the fourth
and fifth niyamas. Should the required study be of the Vedic writings,
of the basic yoga scriptures, or of the guru's own oral instruction?
There are as many replies to these questions as there are ashrams, even
though all agree on the fact that the study must be a virtue, which is
to say, practiced by the novice in a state of perfect humility and re-

ceptivity. It is a matter of forcing one's mind to accept without argument what is taught (and the literature delights in stories of unfortunate novices put to the test by gurus obliging them to accept absurd propositions). As for the virtue of devotion, that also gives rise to considerable divergences of opinion. The bhakti-yoga masters naturally stress religious devotion proper (as did Ramakrishna, who considered worship of the goddess Kali to be a necessary precondition of a yoga apprenticeship); others hold that Ishvara (God) remains passive once he has presided over the creation of a cosmos, so that there is no occasion to worship him in any practical sense. That being so, the virtue of devotion is to be exercised in relation to the guru. But here again, it is not the object of the devotion that is of primary importance but rather the exercise of a mental discipline intended to contribute to the erasing of vasanas.

The texts also give indications of the obstacles to be avoided, many of them the result of the virtues themselves when practiced without discernment. The *Shiva-Samhita* explains, for example, at the beginning of its fifth chapter, that the pleasure that is to be found in studying the *Veda* is as dangerous as that which tempts us to love "women, soft beds, richly decorated cushions" (5.3). Similarly, too much devotion, or even excessive eagerness to practice the higher yoga exercises, bring serious difficulties in their wake. The idea here is that desire (kama) manifests itself in the carrying out of any activity, even those that aim at the very elimination of desire. It is the guru's task to keep watch over the novice's progress and alert him to the dangers of precocious zeal.

Material conditions are no less important. The texts insist that the ashram should be set up in a quiet place with pleasant surroundings, sheltered from the wind and as far as possible from extremes of heat or cold, etc. The idea again is not to allow oneself to be distracted from the single aim, which means one must reduce the irksomeness of daily life to a minimum. If master and disciples do not content themselves with whatever food is offered them, but instead prepare it for themselves (which is particularly the case in the larger and better-known ashrams), then a vegetarian diet is obligatory. The *Hatha-Yoga-Pradipika* specifies that it must consist of "wheat, rice, barley, milk, clarified butter, sugar, honey, ginger, and cucumber" (1.62); it also explains that the yogi will feel better if he eats no more than two-thirds of the amount it would take to sate his hunger. Other texts teach that food should be taken once a day only, the meal to be accompanied by a specific ritual. The reason for this, one need hardly say, is to break the chain of desires on this point too; to eat out of set necessity, at a time fixed in advance, independently of any hunger that may be experienced at any other time, is a method of forcing body and mind into an effective renunciation not merely of gluttony but also of appetite itself as a specific form of concupiscence. If one succeeds, then a particular type of vasanas is attacked and "burned off" by the practitioner's ascesis.

When the master decides that the novice has proved himself to possess the requisite qualities, he confers initiation on him. In some ashrams the ceremony tends to take on a solemn character and may provide an occasion for festivities. More often, however, it remains simple and private. And in any case the structure of the initiation always remains the same: the master adopts his novice, toward whom he will henceforth owe all the duties of a father to a son, and gives him a mantra (a ritual formula), the hearing of which triggers off in some mysterious way the process that is to lead eventually to absolute knowledge.

At the moment of his adoption, the disciple receives a new name, often based upon the guru's intuition of his spiritual son's principal quality. Thus Ramakrishna gave his favorite disciple the name Vivekananda ("he who finds his joy, *ananda,*—in discrimination, *viveka*"), thereby paying tribute to the man's dialectical talent. As for the mantra, that much be communicated secretly: the master whispers it into his disciple's ear, and it is said that the sound waves mingled with the guru's vivifying breath operate a transmutation of the disciple's deep being as he receives them into the most inward part of himself, so that from that very moment his atman begins to play its role as knower with true efficacy. It is said also that certain disciples attain samadhi the instant that their mantra is given them, but in the vast majority of cases the ritual formula is merely a verbal seed that will not come to final fruition until the disciple has recited it, diligently and at length, in accordance with a ritual also laid down by the master (never less than three times a day, and hundreds of times in most cases).

This set recitation is given the name *japa* (repetition). It may be carried out aloud, but a low murmur "like the humming of a bee" is considered to be more efficacious, and mental recitation is even more powerful, albeit reserved for those already far advanced in their yoga apprenticeship.

> By the repetition of the formula
> one gains happiness, here below
> and in the beyond after death;
> one obtains the miraculous powers
> and omnipotence, and joy!
> Received from the guru, the formula
> must be said with great care,
> without haste or lingering,
> with a trusting and attentive heart
> while meditating on its secret.[14]

Every combination of Sanskrit words is capable of constituting a mantra, but usually the guru gives his disciples a simple phrase of a devotional character (e.g., *shri-ganeshaya namah,* "all homage to Ganesha!"). Moreover, many gurus hold that the "secret" of the mantra (and therfore its efficacy) resides more in the "symbolic value" of its phonemes than in the worldly (i.e., accessible to the noninitiate) meaning of the Sanskrit phrase. Many mantras have no appreciable meaning at all, and large numbers consist merely of one syllable. When we come to deal with Tantrism, we shall have occasion to delve further into the (esoteric) theory of the mantra; for the moment, suffice it to say that the mantra par excellence is the syllable *om,* one that is without any profane meaning whatever (it is never used in everyday conversation) but is nevertheless heavy with a symbolism that contains the entire substance of Hindu ideology in condensed form. However, *om* is never given as a mantra to the disciple undergoing initiation, since its use is obligatory for all Hindus, even those who have not renounced the world. It begins and ends any recitation of a sacred text (which means that it is very extensively used in the daily liturgy), and, during japa, *om* is pronounced before every repetition of the specific mantra itself. For instance, in the example given above, the complete formula is: *om shri-ganeshaya namah.*

Once duly initiated, the disciple immediately begins his apprenticeship in the third and fourth stages of yoga, the first of those that are truly specific to it. As we have seen, these involve postures (asanas, "ways of sitting") and breath control (pranayama, "mastery over inhaled air"). In both cases (though the two stages are in fact learned simultaneously) it is a question of attaining perfect mastery over the body, whose intrinsic harmony—unfortunately veiled in the average man—will then be revealed. Patanjali defines what this posture should be in two words: *sthira-sukha*, "firm and relaxed."[15] He feels no necessity to say more than that; primarily because the postures cannot be learned from written texts, but also because those two adjectives on their own sufficiently convey the fact that any position at all is suitable for the practice of yoga, provided it can be held for a long time without discomfort. This is worth stressing; here in the West the word "yoga" inevitably conjures up the image of a man sitting cross-legged, and Europeans imagine that it is impossible to practice yoga without contorting one's limbs in some strange way. What we forget is that this cross-legged position is so dear to Indian yogis quite simply because it is the one that every Indian assumes instinctively on any occasion when we would sit down on a chair—to eat, to read, to rest, to chat with friends. For this reason certain contemporary masters,[16] when teaching yoga to Westerners, ask their students to make themselves comfortable in any way they choose while meditating, in an armchair, on their bed, no matter where, since it is perfectly obvious that the aim of yoga is not physical education but samadhi, which is the result of transcendental meditation.

That said, it must be admitted that our way of holding ourselves is an unnatural one. By sitting on a chair we force our bodies into a zigzag position that is bad for the spine, compresses the abdomen, etc. Observation of people sitting down makes the discomfort of such a posture apparent immediately; they fidget constantly in an attempt to relieve the strain on their muscles and to achieve a comfortable balance. Sitting cross-legged, on the other hand, provides a stable foundation, so that if one is careful to keep one's back straight the spine is always stretched to its true length (whereas we usually let it collapse into itself, with such distressing and now widely recognized results). After a little practice most people can hold this posture without effort, so that it quickly becomes natural. And the texts are categorical on this point: as soon as one is capable of taking up one's preferred asana instinctively, without thinking about it, then one has successfully completed the third stage of classical yoga.

The phrase "cross-legged," of course, is very vague and has no equivalent in India, where several distinct positions, all of which we would have to call "cross-legged," coexist. The yoga manuals vary somewhat in both the names they give these postures and their descriptions of them. To restrict ourselves to the most classical of these asanas —"seated, with legs crossed"—there are the *padma-asana* (lotus position—see figure 4), the *svastika-asana* (position of the auspicious sign —the swastika), the *siddha-asana* (position of perfect being—see figure 5). The lotus, the position most frequently employed by Indian yogis, consists, according to the *Yoga-Kundalini Upanishad* (1.5), in

> *sitting cross-legged,*
> *with the soles of the feet upward*
> *resting on the two thighs;*
> *right foot on left thigh,*
> *left foot on right thigh;*
> *this position, called "the lotus,"*
> *is a remedy for every sickness.*

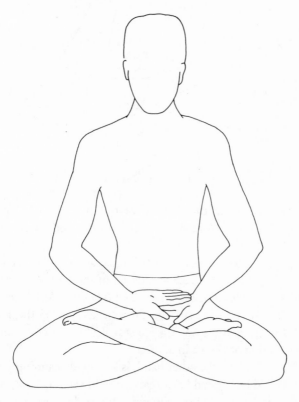

Fig. 4
The padma-asana

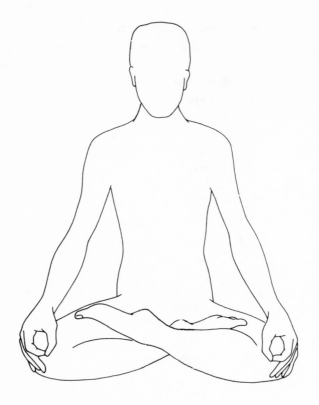

Fig. 5
The siddha-asana

Nothing is said about the position of the arms. Usually they are allowed to hang down toward the knees with fingers interlocked in any way preferred.

The auspicious sign is a variant of the lotus: according to the *Hatha-yoga-Pradipika* (1.19), the feet are placed in the hollows formed by the bent legs, at the level of the knees. The *Gheranda Samhita* (2.13) is no more explicit, particularly as far as the soles of the feet are concerned. But generally speaking the svastika-asana does seem to be an "easy" variation of the padma.

The siddha-asana, on the other hand, is a more demanding posture: both heels should be pressed hard against the lower abdomen, slightly above the genitals; in addition, although the body must remain perfectly straight, the head should be bent forward so that the chin rests

on the chest; the arms hang down so that the back of the hands touch
the knees with fingers curled upwards.

There are many more positions for the practitioner who requires
them: the hatha-yoga treatises give dozens (and mention several hundred not described); but as soon as we leave the basic "cross-legged"
model and its variants, we are entering the domain of acrobatics, and
it is obvious that this means losing view of yoga's single goal, which is
that of achieving samadhi by meditation. For example, there is the
shirsha-asana (see figure 6), which consists in maintaining an upright
position balanced on one's head, arms bent at the elbow to maintain
one's balance, feet together and stretched toward heaven. What do
the texts tell us about this posture? That it ensures good irrigation of
the brain and prevents the hair going white (some even claim that
white hair will become black again as a result of practicing it regularly!). Clearly we are dealing here with an adventitious exercise that
can have a beneficent effect on the yogi's health but which is not, properly speaking, part of yoga technique in the full sense of the term,
since there can evidently be no question of meditating normally and
for long periods in this position.

After all, the *Yoga-Sutras,* and the most important yoga texts based
on them, stress the fact that the postures are not an end in themselves
but intended as a means of facilitating breath control (pranayama).
This later, according to the *Yoga-Sutras* (2.49), consists in "interruption of the process of inhalation and exhalation when in a yoga
posture." From the outset, then, we find the notions of taming, mastery,
control, and beyond these that of total cessation, to which there is
also added the idea of a hierarchic progression, since pranayama is
never exercised until one has learned how to maintain a yoga posture.
The whole ideology of yoga is to be found concentrated in such phrases,
brief though they may be.

In India, ordinary breathing is conceived of as a threefold process.
It consists of inhalation, a pause, then exhalation. Moreover emphasis
is placed on the fact that the individual-in-the-world, because he is
subject to the laws of existence, is incapable of maintaining a stable
respiratory rhythm: at certain times the rate speeds up or slows down
as a result of circumstances external to the breathing itself (running,
anxiety, sleep); moreover, the central pause is reduced to its most simple expression, to the point of being scarcely perceptible, even though

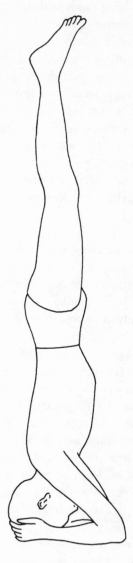

Fig. 6
The shirsha-asana

it is this pause that makes life possible by enabling the body to feed off the energy contained in the inhaled air. The individual living in the world, however, being distracted from himself by his appetites and passions, has no awareness of the functioning of his organs, with the

result that his body can snatch only that amount of the vital nourishment it needs to maintain a precarious existence.

The reader will probably have been struck by the terms "vital energy," "nourishment," and so on, which always make their appearance
as soon as the subject of breathing arises in the Hindu tradition. For
yoga (and in a general way for all the darshanas that deal with it),
breath represents life itself in its most concrete form. So what we are
faced with is a doctrine comparable to the equally traditional Western
belief, current until quite recently, that soul and breath are one and
the same thing. Of course, the Indian tradition does not identify atman
(soul) with prana (breath) in quite that way, but it does hold that
breath is our vital energy (dynamic existence) in the same way that
the atman is pure, impassive essence. Because it holds this view, the
tradition has a natural repugnance to thinking that human existence
is a slave to the atmospheric substance; it prefers to think that we all
receive a "vital breath" at birth, and that the function of respiration is to
circulate it through the body. Thus, the air we inhale is rather to be
thought of as a stimulant, or a vehicle, and the prana is compared to a
fire being fanned into new life by every inhalation: the flame burns
higher, devours the fuel brought in from outside by air and food, then
expels the waste (the "ashes") in the forms of exhaled air and bodily
excretions (sweat, urine, feces).

Clearly, we are a long way here from a simple theory of oxidization;
particularly if we are to believe the texts when they claim that respiration acts above all on our psychic life. We even find statements such as
this one from the *Shiva-Samhita* (3.58 and 3.61):

> By control of the breath,
> one gradually destroys all the karman
> accumulated during previous existences;
> one acquires miraculous powers;
> one moves freely
> throughout the three worlds!

Nor is it by chance that the word *prana* (which corresponds exactly
to the Latin *plenum*) signifies primarily "fullness." As a result of erroneous analysis, it was thought that the basic verbal root involved
was *an* (to blow), and names for other forms of breathing were constructed on this model, such as *apana* (exhaled breath), *vyana* (diffused
breath), *samana* (collected breath), *udana* (ascending breath). Ulti-

mately, though, it is of little importance exactly what is meant by these terms—which the *Yoga-Darshana* texts employ relatively little—the essential point being that the doctrine rests on the unity (the fullness) of the vital breath, analogous in its own domain to the atman, since breath is at the center of bodily activity in the same way as the atman is at the center of the human composite envisaged in its metaphysical totality.

The aim of pranayama is thus to control the energy released by breathing. In fractional terms this control takes the form of a progressive deceleration of the respiratory rhythm, achieved on the one hand by prolonging both inhalation and exhalation, and on the other (and above all) by increasing the central pause to its maximum. In practice it is on this latter development that all the yogi's efforts are brought to bear. The operation called either *ghata* (pot, jar), or more frequently *kumbhaka* (same meaning), consists in holding the inhaled air for as long as possible in the vessel provided by the thorax (except that yoga texts usually refer to the practitioner's abdomen, since it is accepted that the breath reaches down that far). Western observers, such as Dr. Théodore Brosse in 1930,[17] have measured the duration of the kumbhaka and established that the best yogis were able to hold their breath, and thus suspend respiration altogether, for several minutes, thereby establishing conditions that normally result in death (or cause irreversible damage to the brain); and it is this amazing ability that clearly provided the basis of the "living burial" experiments. It should be added, however, that apparently no one has ever been able to record a period of more than five minutes without respiration (and five minutes is an amazing span), while those who did achieve such feats fell into cataleptic states.

The most celebrated masters refuse to indulge in such theatrical demonstrations, which they denounce as pernicious both for the yogi who lends himself to them (he is suspected of having a "desire—a major sin—for self-glorification") and for the spectators (who will acquire a false impression from them of what yoga is). One cannot imagine Ramakrishna, Ramana Maharshi, or Aurobindo making such a spectacle of themselves, either in a public place or in a laboratory.

In order to explain breath control fully, one ought really to go into the theory of the *nadis* (channels of the subtle body) and the repercussions of the exercises on the yogi's personality (particularly insofar as they affect his progress toward samadhi and a realization of the supreme identity). For reasons of method, however, I shall keep my explanation of these things for the fourth section of this book, which deals with Tantric yoga. It will become apparent then how the awakening of the inward energy, the *kundalini,* occurs as a result of pranayama during deep meditation. For the moment, it must be remembered that yamas, niyamas, asanas, and pranayama all have in common the fact that they are violent exercises with the sole purpose of disciplining the body (instincts, bodily agitation, breathing) in order to render it serene, calm, motionless, and collected. Only then will it be able to make use to the highest possible degree of the mental energy that will now have to be "dissolved" in its turn in order to attain samadhi.

8. Dissolving the Mind

T he sole aim of yoga postures and breath control, as we have seen, is not the accomplishment of athletic feats but the realization of a precise objective: mastery over the body. For the yogi it is a question of reaching the point at which he can "forget" the body's existence or, in other words, reduce it to the role of a machine functioning of itself, without any intervention of the consequence (the *chitta,* whose activity, you will remember, yoga makes it an aim to destroy). Indeed, even if, by the end of his novitiate, the adept has succeeded in extinguishing in himself the basis of the desires by which the average man is enslaved (that being the sole object of the restraints and spiritual disciplines), he still remains subject to other desires: those that take the form, in all of us, of corporeal agitation and unrhythmical breathing, together with all the consequences these things infallibly have upon our personalities as a whole. The progression is clear: yamas and niyamas deal with what one might term the elementary vasanas[1] (those that concern everyday behavior: concupiscence/generosity, lying/veracity, etc.), and constitute a "moral" discipline that is clearly essential to anyone entering upon the hard road of yoga but still not sufficient to ensure the attainment of samadhi. The novice who succeeds (not without a struggle) in "behaving well" is, after all, no more than a man who has proved his force of character; yoga is not a school of social conduct (we have already seen that in one sense it is the negation of dharma). To go further along the path the yogi must then go through a second major stage, one that consists, as we have seen, in taming his body's vital energies. Once he has succeeded in this, he is no longer in danger of being distracted by the constant and insistent demands made upon us by our bodies. A sort of muscular and respiratory peace invades the man who practices asanas and pranayama, replacing the perpetual war between "flesh and spirit" that is the lot of most living beings.

However, even when one is motionless (in a position that has become so natural that one no longer remembers ever having consciously learned it) and one's breathing has been disciplined to the point of transmutation into pure rhythmic harmony, this still does not mean that all distraction has ceased. Quite the contrary, in fact; the texts seem to take delight in pointing out that distraction actually increases to a quite considerable extent, both in quality (it becomes more insistent) and in quantity (one's curiosity extends to a much larger number of objects). As the mind is freed from a large part of the solicitations to which it was formerly accustomed ("ordinary" desires, responses to bodily demands), so our senses acquire a proportionately superior efficiency, since the physiological serenity achieved permits them to be used to the full. One sees better, hears better, and so on, because the mental organ can devote itself entirely to sifting the information being fed to it by eyes, skin, tongue, nose, or ears. So the physical serenity and immobility acquired by pranayama and asanas put a stop to the wastage of mental effort hitherto necessitated by continual psychomotor responses to the incessant demands of a body enslaved to agitation. The next step, therefore, is to deal with the sense organs themselves, and to achieve a similar cessation of the fantasmagoria of "sensual" (in the broadest sense) images characteristic of mental life. The motionless yogi seated in the lotus position, breathing slowly, would be no more than a ridiculous daydreamer if he simply allowed his thoughts to go wandering off into the outside world. The slightest sound, the most fleeting visual stimulus, the faintest scent in the air would trigger off tempests of the imagination fueled by the impregnations (vasanas) in which his mind is so thoroughly steeped.

The fifth stage of yoga, then, according to the itinerary laid down by Patanjali,[2] is that of *pratyahara* (withdrawal or abstraction of the senses). To help us understand exactly what is involved here, the texts at our disposal like to employ the image of the tortoise, which is capable of drawing its legs and head back into itself when it so desires. The Indian conception of how our sense organs function is in fact similar to that of our own classical antiquity. Like the Greeks, the Hindus believe that organs such as the eye or ear function as though they possess some kind of mysterious antennae, extensions of themselves that reach out to touch the objects which engage our attention. In other words, our eyes do not receive light impressions but, on the contrary, emit a kind of beam that reconnoiters the outside world for us and, as it were, "caresses it with our gaze." Here again, we are dealing with one of the essential characteristics of Indian thought, which attributes a dynamic value and a power of radiation to every manifestation of life. And it is precisely this process of externalization, of dispersion, that yoga attempts to destroy—a goal that makes it, as we have said, profoundly antinatural (at least from the Indian point of view) since it is doing violence to the normal functioning of the human composite. Needless to say, the principal aim is always the same: to suppress one after the other all one's bodily mechanisms in order to free the mind from external solicitations.

The yogi must therefore practice cutting off all contact with the world by "closing the windows" of his body. That is easily said; but even though one closes one's eyelids, keeps one's hands closed, slows down one's breathing, there still remain the light impressions received through the eyelids, the skin still goes on feeling warmth and cold, the nose still smells any scent borne on the air inhaled, however faint it may be. And what about the sense of hearing? How is one to prevent oneself hearing, even if one refuses to listen? The difficulty of such an undertaking is evident. And when it comes to describing the method to be employed the texts prove particularly discreet, not out of any desire for concealment, but because we have now entered a domain in which the essential cannot be reached except by personal practice combined with theoretical instruction from one's guru.[3] The latter will do his best to foster in his disciple a conscious awareness of the fact that his senses are not purely automatic functions but "forces," "sovereign powers," called in Sanskrit *indriyas* or *devatas*.

The choice of these terms is highly significant: *indriya,* in the *Veda,* denotes the forces at the disposal of Indra, king of the gods, in his task of governing the world, while *devata* (from *deva,* "god") signifies "divinity" or "deity," and usually denotes the lesser gods who act as assistants to the major gods. Thus Varuna, guardian of the cosmic order, is helped by innumerable "spies" (the Vedic rishis call them *spashah*) whose task it is to hunt out infringements of dharma and carry out the sentences that Varuna then pronounces on those responsible. The Maruts, Indra's band of followers, who assist him in his function as universal sovereign, are termed in mythological language— along with many other members of the pantheon—devatas, meaning subsidiary deities in the service of a major god, or external manifestations of his intrinsic power, if one prefers to use a metaphysical vocabulary. Indra's function is to overcome the forces hostile to dharma by violent means, and the Maruts are the "soldiers" he employs in his battles. But in fact, even the most ancient Brahmanic theology has always preferred to say that the god himself is the incarnation of this beneficent violence and that the minor deities who assist him are its concrete, dynamic expression in the sphere of things. Here one recognizes the characteristic Hindu notion of "power." At once cosmic forces and true deities (that is, playing a mythological role), the indriyas are not quite divine individuals yet not quite mere mechanical reactions either; they enjoy a certain freedom of maneuver (while remaining always subject to the god of whom they are extensions) and yet can be disbanded at any time like regiments on the decision of the high command.

The complexity and the paradox of this situation reflect the way Hindu tradition interprets the workings of perception and motor responses to sensorial stimuli: what we take to be a system of automatic effects is really just the result of the average man's indifference—or, to be more accurate, of his distraction. Our eyes and ears are left permanently in the "on" position, as it were, but like good servants of an inattentive master they are left to their own devices to function as best they can. As a result, the servants soon usurp the directive function themselves: they alone are truly active, and the incessant buzzing of their zealous activity finally lulls asleep a mind already predisposed by its nature to idleness. If we accept this view, then the program of yoga becomes self-evident: to restore to the mind its rightful directive function, so that it is able to force its indriyas to cease their activity. And if he does succeed in bringing about this change within himself, then clearly the adept will have made it possible to employ the intrinsic power of his manas (mind, thought) to the full, now that it has at last been aroused from its lethargy. It is thus the mental organ itself that must be employed to achieve pratyahara: the "withdrawal of the senses" is a matter of will.

Following on from this the texts usually say that breath control automatically produces a tendency in the mind to fix its attention on a single point (Vyasa, commentary on the *Yoga-Sutras,* 2.53). And this *ekagrata* or "sustained attention directed onto one point or object" is indeed the natural consequence of an apprenticeship in pranayama, since the very difficulty of that exercise demands unfailing mental concentration, rather like that of an artisan putting all his energy into an absorbing task. It is a well-known fact that at such moments we allow ourselves to be distracted far less easily by external solicitations: the mental organ has the indriyas well under control and is screening the information they are sending in. In other words, it is acting as a censor and deciding whether that information from the indriyas is worthy of its attention or whether it should be ignored. We must all know at least one story like that of the mathematician who, deep in thought, was taking a stroll through Paris when he found himself confronted by the back of a hansom cab. The surface of stretched black cloth presented itself to him as an ideal blackboard, and so, pulling a piece of chalk from his pocket, he started writing the data of the problem that was preoccupying him on the cloth, wholly unaware of anything untoward in his actions. When the cab drove off, the mathematician was seen running after it so as not to interrupt the development of his equations. That is what yogis mean by *ekagrata*. Not intellectual "absent-mindedness," wandering "with its head in the clouds," but the very opposite: an attentive functioning of the mental organ as it concentrates all its power onto a single object.

Mark you, our mathematician had not achieved a "withdrawal of the senses"; his hand still felt the texture of the chalk, his ear could hear the sarcastic remarks of the passers-by, his eyes did perceive the movement of the cab away from him, etc. Yet the fact that he was able to act as he did shows that he possessed a habit of mental concentration sufficiently strong to cause him to neglect, for a short while at least, the indications provided by his sensorial organs; his mind decided (even though it was without any clear awareness on his part) that it was of minimal importance that the "blackboard" was in fact the back of a hansom cab. This gives a good idea of how the simple practice of ekagrata leads to effective control of the indriyas by the mental organ (manas). And yet that control remains precarious, fleeting, and above all incomplete, since sensorial information continues to be received and is thus capable of distracting the mind (so that the mathematician only ran a few yards in fact before being "called to order" by his mind as it yielded to the pressure of its indriyas and accepted their warnings). Whereas, if one succeeds in imposing true silence on one's sense organs, then one seals oneself off totally from the outside world, and the possibility of distraction caused by outside intervention disappears.

The yogi therefore practices ekagrata by concentrating all his powers of attention on the correct realization of pranayama, "breath control." In doing this he is conditioning his mind so that it is in the correct state for his apprenticeship in sense withdrawal: the rest is a matter of willpower and steady perseverance. And of endurance too, since it goes without saying that pratyahara must be practiced in "heroic" fashion, or in other words for longer and longer periods in order to achieve ever greater and greater proficiency. The *Shiva Samhita,* for example, states that the yogi cannot claim to have passed through the stage of pratyahara (the fifth of yoga's eight rungs) until he is able to maintain sense withdrawal for three hours at a stretch. However, it must be added that this same work, and in the same context (3.67 to 70), also states that the breath should be held, simultaneously, for the same length of time (eight *dandas,* or 192 minutes). This is a far cry from the few minutes ordinarily recommended for the kumbhaka (retention of inhaled breath). It is therefore clear that sense withdrawal falls into that category of yoga exercises about which there is nothing that Western observers can usefully say; physiologically, according to the scientific criteria we accept and apply, a kumbhaka of such duration is impossible to achieve. And if it were possible, even for a shorter time, the yogi would fall into a coma, a state in which sense withdrawal would certainly become very complete indeed —for obvious reasons! So let us simply make this one more opportunity for emphasizing the rift that has existed now for several centuries at least between the exact sciences and traditional teachings.

To return to pratyahara itself: it must now be explained that the indriyas are not destroyed but merely lulled to sleep when sense withdrawal becomes effective, and since they are still alive (life being a condition of existence), that sleep reduces their activity but does not wholly negate it. Patanjali and Vyasa explain that their activity in this state is similar to that of the mind itself when in a state of ekagrata. We read in the *Yoga-Sutras* (2.54) that "when the sensory faculties turn away from objects, they function in imitation of attentive thought"; which Vyasa, in his commentary on this passage, further elucidates by means of an image: "Just as, when a queen bee flies off, the other bees fly off also in her train, and swarm when she alights, so do the indriyas fix themselves when thought does so." What is involved is clearly just another mode of attention rather than a new and different phenomenon. Sense withdrawal seems therefore to be a means rather than an end (as indeed, every step in yoga is a function of every other step, especially of those that precede it).

In other words, the aim of sense withdrawal is to prepare the mind for the next stage of yoga, the one Patanjali calls dharana or "mental concentration" and which, he says, consists in maintaining the mind fixed in a single direction (*Yoga-Sutras,* 3.1). The difficulty here lies in the distinction between ekagrata (intense attention) and the mental concentration of dharana, since it is indisputable that attention may be held to be a form of mental concentration, and vice versa. Nevertheless, if we take the context into account, then the difference between them will become clear without any need for extensive explanations. Since yoga, like all Hinduism's traditional disciplines, is a continuous progress, we can be sure that dharana is in some sense "higher" (that is, more intense, more efficacious) than ekagrata. Where the latter was merely the fixing of mental activity onto a single object, dharana must appear as a motionless meditation, a silent collecting together of the mind's powers. Remember that, whenever the breath is held (kumbhaka), the attention tends to become fixed of its own accord, even if it be merely on the act of breath control itself, which does in fact require undistracted thought if the exercise is to be correctly carried out. That is ekagrata. Further, when the adept has succeeded in achieving sense withdrawal, his attention is necessarily improved, since all unwanted external solicitations cease. Nevertheless, thought continues to exist and therefore to live. As we know, life for the Hindu tradition must imply activity, diffusion, dispersion, multiplicity, etc.

In other words, ekagrata (even when enriched by pratyahara) can never be perfect; attention no more entails the dissolution of mental activity than a correct yoga posture abolishes corporeal life. On the contrary, with the body already immobile and respiration suspended (or extremely decelerated), mental activity actually attains its maximum efficiency when freed in addition from the constraints entailed by sensory activity. It is at this moment that the individual thinks best, that his brain functions with greatest east and accuracy, because the intuitions emanating from the buddhi (intelligence)—no longer obscured by the smokescreen of impulses arising from sensory information and the vasanas impregnating them—become more easily perceptible. The mind opens itself up to them and is able to absorb ever more and more intellectual light. The *Amritanada Upanishad* (1.14ff) describes the process like this:

> *By it, one gains serenity;*
> *one sees forms*
> *as the blind man sees them,*
> *one hears sounds*
> *as the deaf man hears them,*
> *and the body is no longer anything*
> *but a block of wood!*
> *Yes, practicing dharana*
> *is to recognize, by reflection,*
> *that thought is molded*
> *by desire and intention,*
> *and it is to constrain thought*
> *to be attentive to the soul alone,*
> *till it is united with it!*

Which means that, thanks to pranayama, and to ekagrata, which proceeds naturally from it, the mental organ finds itself quieted (*shanta*) as a result of practicing sense withdrawal. From then on, if it sees forms, if it hears sounds, those forms and sounds cannot be anything but fantasms arising from memory, constructions of the fancy colored by the yogi's mental impregnations (vasanas). And since they lack any material basis, these false perceptions resemble those of the blind or the deaf: they have intense existence, but only as manifestations of "pure" mental activity, in other words mental activity functioning on its own, in a closed circuit. Ultimately, our consciousness of the life of our body (which continues even when that body is motionless and "quieted") is annihilated: the body becomes an inert thing, a block of wood. And it is at this point that the yogi, concentrating the entire force of his mental organ on this single object, compels his thought to turn back upon itself until it is knowing its true nature (and we know that knowing in the Hindu tradition is something very different from mere profane knowledge). Through such turning back upon itself, the mind acquires a conscious awareness of the role played by desire (kama) in its functioning, and simultaneously realizes that the only way of freeing itself from the bondage of desire is to have recourse to the atman, which, being situated beyond the existential sphere, is unaffected by any vasana and therefore enjoys pure freedom. Once the mind has "recognized" its true condition, the only goal the individual can conceivably set himself is union with that pure freedom. Such a union, of course, cannot actually be effected until the yogi reaches the last yoga stage of all: samadhi. Dharana, the sixth stage, constitutes the yogi's preparation for that union, the stage at which he finally catches sight of his goal, senses it within his grasp.

It goes without saying that dharana necessitates a long apprenticeship; the yogi is invited to attempt progressively more and more difficult sorts of meditation. It is said, for example, that meditation should begin by taking beings or things belonging to the tangible world as its object. They are not really seen, heard, or touched, of course, since the senses have by now ceased to fulfill their functions: the objects are merely mental constructions. At a later stage one meditates on the gods; later still on metaphysical subjects (particularly on the atman, brahman, their intrinsic oneness, etc.) At each level a precise method is given for contructing the mental image that is to provide the foundation for the meditation. For example, if the yogi decides to fix his thought on an image of Vishnu, then he must build that image up progressively. Instead of giving himself a total vision all at once, he must fashion his Vishnu-object piece by piece, like a conscientious craftsman, beginning from the bottom (the cushion on which Vishnu is seated, the position of his feet, the color of his garment, etc.), then gradually working upward (vision of the head, eyes, forehead, crown encircling the god's head, etc.). Eventually the moment will come when the mind reaches the central point around which the entire image is organized (which may be Vishnu's third eye, or another god's glowing heart, or the light emanating from his head, etc.), and, from that instant on, the vision becomes total, so that the yogi receives an intuition of the essential truth (atman/brahman) of which the image he has been building was merely an exterior form. In this way he reaches the goal he had initially set himself: meditation upon the soul.

Using the same method, the yogi may mentally draw a mandala,[4] employing all his powers of concentration and assiduity to produce an almost infinite complexity of detail. As though working on a kind of puzzle, he slots the various elements into their allotted places, one by one, until the desired image is finally complete and he is able to insert the central point around which it is organized. This is another

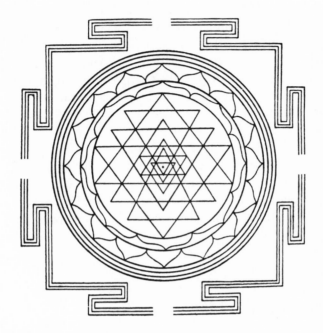

Fig. 7
A mandala: the shri-yantra

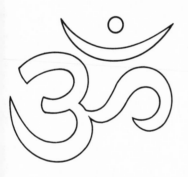

Fig. 8
The syllable *om*

moment at which he intuitively grasps the metaphysical meaning of the diagram he has constructed; he sees in it the magical richness of the phenomenal world blossoming from the central geometric point (i.e., a point without thickness, color, form, etc.) that symbolizes atman/brahman. It is significant that the other Sanskrit word denoting this kind of diagram is *yantra*. Derived as it is from the verb root *yam* (to tame or master), this term clearly indicates that the mandala is essentially a "method of taming" (the primary meaning of *yantra*), a tool for forcing the mind to perform the maneuver of turning back upon itself that will enable it to see the path to the essential unity beyond existential multiplicity (see figure 7).

The syllable *om* also lends itself to the same use. One can meditate upon it either by "hearing" (mentally) its sound or else by visualizing it in graphic form. In either case the process is similar to the one just described: the details are inserted into their correct place, one after the other, until the insertion of the final point that triggers the total, synthetic intuition of the mystery. In graphic form, *om* looks not unlike our figure three with the addition of a downward curving tail with an upturned crescent containing a dot (the *bindu,* which is the graphic representation of essence) floating over it (see figure 8). As a sound, *om* can be broken down into three elements: the two vowels *a* and *u*—which in accordance with the rules of Sanskrit phonetics become *o* when combined—and the resonant nasal sound represented by *m,* which is prolonged with a kind of fermata (represented in the graphic form by the *bindu*). As the *Dhyanabindu Upanishad* (1.18) tells us:

> *All-permeating as oil*
> *poured in an unbroken stream,*
> *or as the constant reverberation*
> *of a bell ringing in the distance,*
> *is the indescribable resonance*
> *of the syllable* om:
> *he who knows it knows the Veda.*

Moreover, the knowledge acquired by meditating on the syllable *om* during the exercise of dharana is not only higher than that obtained by a study of the scriptures (the *Veda* as the *Upanishad* put it), it is also indistinguishable from the vision of the Lord seen by "the heart's eye" that all yogis seek:

> *At the center of the calyx*
> *of the heart's lotus*
> *it holds itself motionless,*
> *shining like a lamp*
> *that never goes out;*
> *it is upon it that one must meditate,*
> *the syllable* om,
> *in which must be recognized*
> *the Lord himself . . .*[5]

The symbolic wealth of *om* (a single syllable but made up of three elements, uniting in itself both existential multiplicity and the unity of essence, etc.) and the high place allotted to it by yoga theoreticians become apparent in their concern to show that the creative Word (ultimately identical with the Absolute) resides in the heart of every creature. The fourth section of this book will devote several pages to an exposition of the symbolism of *om,* but for the moment it is enough to say that meditation on the primordial sound (*nada*) is given clear precedence by the texts, presumably because the visual mandala is felt by the masters to be excessively static when compared with the auditory effect of the formal monosyllable. Because the latter is a continuous, eternal vibration (*amrita-nada*) it is perceived as dynamic in essence. And as we know, the notions of radiating energy and movement are fundamental in Hinduism to any representation of the blossoming, unfurling world of phenomena, with the result that *om* is also frequently compared to the sun, which as we saw earlier is another customary image for the same vital force:

> *Like ten million suns,*
> om *shines perpetually*
> *at the heart of all men:*
> *that is why its power must be used*
> *to gather the breath within one*
> *until one attains the complete disappearance*
> *of all other sound.*[6]

The aim of meditation on *om,* or upon any other "support" (mandala, divine image, etc.), is, as the *Upanishad* says, the total disappearance of any other thought: the yogi's mind must no longer be anything but the hearing of *om.* Better still, the mind must be totally annihilated by a global apprehension of the atman in the form of a single synthetic perception in which the sound heard, the light seen, the taste savored, etc., are all commingled (because the Absolute is also symbolically represented as the *rasa* or savor of all things, or as the scent—that is to say the essence—of the universe).

It is clear, therefore, that pratyahara has in no way destroyed the senses but rather "gathered them together," concentrated them in the individual's inmost recesses so that they become able to taste, hear, see, touch, feel the only "thing" worthy of attention: atman. Similarly, mental activity is not abolished by dharana but fixed upon the only object of reflection worthy of it: the supreme identity, that of atman and brahman. In order to be effective and salutary, this mental fixation should lead to the dissolution of the mind itself, at least in its conscious form:

> *When he has tamed his mind,*
> *when he is detached from everything,*
> *the yogi is indifferent*
> *to all that is not the sound;*
> *renouncing all exercise of his mind*
> *on any other thing but his atman;*
> *thanks to meditation he dissolves*
> *his mind in* pranava.[7]

The terms employed by the *Upanishad* here are particularly significant in this context: *nade chittam viliyate* ("the consciousness is dissolved in the sound"). In a sense, then, one might say that perfect dharana does effectively realize the aim of yoga, since that aim, according to the *Yoga-Sutras* themselves (1.2), is nothing other than the dissolution of mental activity (*yogash chittavritti-nirodhah*). And some schools do in fact teach that the final step has been taken once the yogi has succeeded in dissolving his mind into an inner hearing of the syllable *om* (together with the inward vision of its light, etc.). Hence the term *laya-yoga* (the yoga of dissolution) used by some masters. The *Kshurika Upanishad* (1.24ff) asserts, for example:

> *When the knife*
> *of the fixed mind*
> *whetted by breath control,*
> *sharpened on the stone of renunciation*
> *has cut through the weave of life,*
> *the adept is forever*
> *released from his bonds.*
> *Freed from all desire,*
> *he becomes immortal;*
> *delivered from temptations,*
> *having cut through the toils of existence*
> *he is no longer in samsara.*

It is remarkable to find a text stating so categorically, despite the teaching of the *Yoga-Sutras,* the idea that dharana (fixing of the

mind), prepared by pranayama (breath control) and samnyasa (renunciation), is the knife (*kshurika,* hence the name of this *Upanishad*)
that cuts the toils of the net holding the soul captive:

> *As a bird,*
> *imprisoned by a net,*
> *will fly up to heaven*
> *after the toils are cut,*
> *so the adept's soul,*
> *released from the bonds of desire,*
> *by the knife of yoga,*
> *escapes forever*
> *from the prison of samsara.*[8]

It must be added, however, that the majority of gurus are of the
opinion that dissolution of the mind is rather a condition of liberation
than liberation itself; after his apprenticeship in dharana the adept
has two further stages to master—dhyana and samadhi—before reaching the final goal.

9. Seeing God Face to Face

he yogi must now enter upon the last two stages of his journey. The quest is coming to its end; the Absolute, we may
venture to say, is within arm's length. The yogi has succeeded in taming all the forces of his being one after another—first the instincts, then bodily movement, breathing, the senses,
and mental activity. He has reached the point at which consciousness
(chitta) is dissolved by the practice of dharana; and, as we have just
said, for certain texts this is the ultimate step, since the yoga program
as laid down by the *Yoga-Sutras* has been realized.[1] However, if we
refer back to the schemes of the human composite (figures 1 and 2),
we shall see that beyond the manas (mental organ) there is the buddhi
and also, of course, the atman. That the latter cannot be involved in
yoga as a method of spiritual progress is self-evident, since the Absolute, by definition, cannot be affected by anything at all; but what of
the buddhi? Its position is in itself paradoxical, since it belongs simultaneously to the "corporeal" totality (body, senses, thought) and to
the atman whose light it reflects. The various opposing schools within
yoga as a whole teach either that the buddhi is a true manifestation of
the atman/brahman (hypostasis of the Absolute), or that it is a
higher form of mental activity. In the first case it is imperishable and
continues to transmigrate along with the atman until the moment of
liberation. In the second it remains a transitory epiphenomenon that
the yogi must tame in the same way as he did his body, his breath, and
his thought. The prestige of the buddhi is nevertheless such that even
those who hold it to be "corporeal" hesitate to imagine that it can be
subjected to constraints of any kind. Thus the *Kshurika Upanishad*
(quoted at the end of chapter 8), which identifies dharana ("fixation
of thought") with the end of yoga, prefers to "forget" the buddhi
rather than ask the adept to bend it to his law (and even less to "dissolve" it, an unthinkable notion within the Hindu cultural context).
Moreover, such positions are very rarely expressed, and most texts
retain the program of Patanjali, who follows dharana with dhyana

and samadhi. So that if thought (manas) has been dissolved and the journey is still not over, then clearly there is only the buddhi left to continue it. The reader will recall the image of the chariot: the atman, an unwilling passenger in a chariot (the body) drawn by horses (the indriyas or organs of perception and action) controlled via the reins (the manas) by a driver who is none other than the buddhi itself. It is, in fact, intelligence (Plato's *nous*) that has called the tune from the outset. In obedience to its directives, the body has been stabilized (by the practice of asanas), the indriyas have been "interiorized" (by pratyahara), the mana has been "dissolved" (by dharana), so that now at last the chariot has come to a halt; the moment has arrived when the atman will be able to step out of it—the image of final liberation.

As for the mental impregnations (vasanas), they are progressively "burned off" during the journey. The restraints and spiritual disciplines (yamas and niyamas) had already destroyed a good proportion of them, and now breath control (leading to ekagrata) and above all sense withdrawal and fixation of thought (dharana) have done the rest. Since it was the vasanas that were tarnishing the buddhi's mirror, then, the mirror has been wiped clean of their grime and can at last perform its true role. In other words, now that the yogi has achieved the perfection of dharana, the light of his atman is being perfectly reflected by the inner mirror, the buddhi, and its great spiritual radiance can expand the adept's inner universe into a cosmic brightness. As the stanza, quoted earlier, of the *Kshurika Upanishad* puts it, the immortal light "shines forth like ten million suns!" And yet even this experience is not enough, because the subject/object distinction is still being maintained; the human composite, even when totally under the control of the buddhi, remains distinct from the atman. Although in the presence of pure essence, it is still part of existence itself. It is being bathed in a light exterior to it, like a planet that is being given life by the sun but would become once more a lifeless pebble if the great star happened to be extinguished.

Admittedly, the light emanating from the atman is inextinguishable (it is the *lux perpetua* of the Persian religions, whose symbolism was taken over by Christianity), so that certain yoga practitioners understandably choose to remain content with this situation. Such yogis are recruited mostly from among the followers of bhakti-yoga (the yoga of devotion), whose aim is to achieve a beatific vision of the Lord.

Having succeeded through dharana in opening themselves to the divine light, which is a privileged manifestation of grace, they feel no need to go any further, since they believe that the state of communion with God in which they will henceforth exist is an end in itself. For them, liberation is cohabitation with the divinity until the end of the cosmic cycle. But, as I have had occasion to stress many times already, the program of classical yoga is more ambitious: it is concerned with releasing the soul (jiva-atman, "the living soul") from its captive condition and thereby restoring it to its true status. In Vishnu's paradise, the soul of the bhakta (practitioner of bhakti-yoga) remains incarnate: it continues to exist, by the same token as the Lord himself and the glorious world in which it resides with him. Whatever the perfection of beatitude his contemplation of God attains for him, the adept cannot claim to be truly liberated; he could only be that if he were to leave the existential sphere and return to essence itself. If one wishes to follow the teaching of the *Yoga-Sutras,* it is necessary to go beyond dharana and to travel through the two stages of the journey that still remain.

The first of these two stages is dhyana, a difficult word to translate if we are to avoid confusion with dharana. For the sake of convenience we will keep to "meditation," as do the majority of authors (though you will recall that we have been obliged on some occasions to translate *dharana* too by "meditation"), with an adjective sometimes added to emphasize its "metaphysical" nature (for example, "transcendental meditation"). Other writers prefer "contemplation" or "perfect communion." These varying approximations do at least have the advantage of indicating that dhyana must not be thought of as any ordinary mental operation. Indeed, in the eyes of the yoga masters themselves it could not be, since all mental activity has already been annihilated by the exercise of dharana. It is the buddhi that is operating from now on, and its field of action is located beyond that of ordinary thought, beyond reasoning, and also, needless to say, beyond passion and imagination, since they are the expression of the vasanas destroyed in previous stages. The intelligence is above all intuitive knowing: it is the buddhi that "sees essence," or rather that receives its light. So that if the adept succeeds in using his buddhi at maximum efficiency he will have the possibility, through its agency, of "seeing God face to face," it being understood that in the yoga

world-system (darshana) God is another name for the Absolute, and
that "to see God" is "to become God," to "realize" the fact that the
atman, the essential part of our self, is in no way different from
brahman:

> *And you will also be able to meditate*
> *on Ishana, (the Lord), the truth,*
> *the non-dual knowledge,*
> *pure, eternal, and without past*
> *as well as without present or future;*
> *subtle, inconceivable, unperceivable,*
> *without smell or savor, unmeasurable;*
> *the One that is no other than the soul,*
> *being-consciousness-joy;*
> *realizing: "I am that brahman!"*
> *you will achieve liberation![2]*

You may have noticed that this same text initially seems applicable
to dharana, which could also be "supported" by an inner vision of a
divine image (or a mandala, etc.). However, dhyana does not entail
the progressive building up of the "support" necessary in dharana. It
is given all at once, as "subject" rather than object; so that we are on
a higher level here from the very outset. The meditation on the Lord
(*Ishana* is one of the names of Shiva) described here is a conscious
apprehension (on the spiritual level) of the true nature of God: he
is at the same time the One and the pure knowledge that one can have
of that One; he is the atman and supreme being (sach-chid-ananda;
"being-consciousness-joy"); he is brahman and truth; and to know
that (i.e., to "realize intuitively that one is That") leads to liberation.
The important thing, given such a context, is the adjective "non-dual"
applied to knowledge. It means that the knowledge thus obtained is an
identification that abolishes all difference between knower and known.
And once there is no longer any distinction between subject and object, then one is in the "world of essence"—the supreme goal that the
yogi set himself at the very beginning of his journey.

However, it is only "moments of intuition" that are involved here,
the texts say, rather than any permanent identification (for, if it were
otherwise, the yogi would have reached the end of his journey, and
it is difficult to see what the next stage could possibly consist in).
Some *Upanishads* even go so far as to say the yogi may tire himself out

with this kind of contemplation. In the *Dhyanabindu Upanishad* (1.93), for example, we find:

> *If the inner eye becomes tired*
> *from its contemplation of the soul in the heart,*
> *to rest it one must*
> *use meditation to conjure up*
> *the image of a white circle.*

It is interesting to find that fatigue causes the yogi to descend again to a type of vision resembling the meditation on mandalas that he previously practiced in dharana. But again there is a difference, because the perception of the yantra in dhyana is synthetic, not analytic: the yogi simply intuits a structure (and the simplest possible) without any need to construct it. Furthermore, the same text warns that at this level

> *fantastic images arise*
> *visual and auditory hallucinations,*
> *fantasms of all sorts*
> *that quickly tire the inner eye.*

And when this happens, the remedy is to conjure up a yellow circle, then a red one; serenity then ensues and the fantasms fade away of themselves.

> *The adept must then draw nearer,*
> *gradually, to absolute repose,*
> *by fixing his mind*
> *on the universal soul*
> *by the use of his intelligence . . .*
> *after that he perceives nothing whatever.*

At that point he has reached perfect peace (*shanti*), the absolute repose in which the universal sarvam duhkham ("all is suffering") is annihilated. We read in the *Bhagavad-Gita* (6.19):

> *Just as an oil lamp,*
> *when the wind stops,*
> *burns with a motionless flame,*
> *so the yogi with his mind held still*
> *attains union with his soul.*

Here again the favored images are those of immobility, silence, the extinguishing of vision, etc.—the ones, in fact, that best convey to the Hindu, by their contrast to the agitation and multiplicity of existence, what the return to essence is.

Having dealt with the visual, auditory, and other fantasmagorias that assail the yogi even when he has reached the stage of dhyana, we now come to the celebrated "miraculous powers" acquired by the yoga practitioner when he has reached the highest levels of spiritual experience. The masters do in fact teach that the yogi—as a consequence of his perfect knowledge of his own physiological and psychological chemistry—can provoke reactions within himself that render possible extraordinary physical transformations (change of color, invisibility, etc.), as well as a complete mutation of his fundamental condition of being.

> *Thus he wins the gift of prophecy;*
> *he transports himself, as he wishes,*
> *anywhere in space.*
> *He sees all that is, even at the greatest distances;*
> *he hears all, sees the invisible,*
> *and can enter at will into*
> *the body of another person,*
> *change all metals into gold*
> *by immersing them in his urine;*
> *he can make anything disappear*
> *and fly, if he so wishes, in the air.*[3]

Needless to say, there can be no question of the true yogi's indulging indiscriminately in the use of such superhuman powers. If he did, he would simply be proving that he has not succeeded in annihilating desire within himself, showing that he is still a long way from attaining liberation. All the same, these manifestations of the power acquired by meditation ought not to be wholly neglected. The yogi should experience their use, if only to check that he is not deceiving himself in believing that he has reached such and such a point in his spiritual development. That done, he transcends them and "forgets" them in order to avoid any danger of being distracted from the supreme goal.

In addition to those mentioned in the passage from the *Shiva-*

Samhita quoted above, the powers most frequently cited are: the power to reduce one's body to the size of an atom or to increase it to immense dimensions, the power either to weigh nothing or to become so heavy that one cannot be moved by anyone or anything, and so forth. Leaving the strictly physical plane we find: the power to know the existences one has passed through in previous lives, to read other people's thoughts, to leave one's own body, to levitate, etc. At a higher level one acquires a comprehension of the secrets of nature, metaphysical wisdom, the fulfillment of all desires, etc. The fact that these miraculous manifestations (*vibhuti*) occur on different planes shows that they are in reality the realization, the fulfillment (*siddhi*) of faculties that remain latent in the average man. Indian tradition does not doubt for a moment that everyone has the power to read someone else's mind, send messages through time and space, know the future and the past, rise up into the air, or live for centuries. And though these powers remain inaccessible to the vast majority of human beings, they still exist, and can be awakened in the man who succeeds through yoga in withdrawing himself from the solicitations of the world of senses. In this domain, as in all others, it is concentration of the mind, perfect attention, and meditation that ensure success. But what we must bear in mind is that the use of the terms *vibhuti* (unfurling, manifestation) and *siddhi* (fulfillment, perfection) implies that these powers are not in any way made or created by yoga but merely brought by it to their maximum efficiency. Here again yoga is doing violence to nature, promoting an individual (before his soul has been liberated) to a position of power that carries with it the risk of disruption to society, should enough yogis decide to dally at this stage and enjoy the exploitation of their siddhis.

Which brings us to the fact that the Hindu community as a whole, while respecting the "salutary" doctrine of yoga, nevertheless views with mistrust those that practice it. It has an ill-formulated feeling that these renouncers are defying dharma. Don't they accept people of different castes into their ashrams? Don't they preach deserting one's family, celibacy, scorn for wealth? What if everyone did as they said? What if everyone stopped working and observing the customs? Society would collapse! And what's more, these people are powerful magicians too. They can do things that only genies and gods ought to be able to do. So there is a tendency to regard them as sorcerers, with the result that those sadhus who lack sufficient prestige to become

respected gurus are wise to keep away from villages. Apart from anything else, contact with them defiles any high-caste Hindu; as we
have seen, yogis when begging for their food must take great care not
to touch those who give them alms. Moreover, the possibility that they
might start exploiting their miraculous powers can only accentuate the
fear with which the average man regards these extraordinary beings.
Therefore:

> *He shall not seek for these powers,*
> *and if he has them will not glory in them*
> *if he wishes to be a true yogi.*
> *Very much to the contrary, keeping them secret,*
> *he will act in the world*
> *as though he were an ordinary man,*
> *or even a simpleton,*
> *not to say a deaf-mute.*
> *Indeed, people ask so many questions*
> *that if the adept wanted to answer them*
> *he would lose sight of his own way of life*
> *which is to move forward along his road*
> *without interesting himself in the world.*[4]

It would be impossible to remind yoga practitioners more firmly that
the important thing is to maintain one's progress along one's spiritual
itinerary (the "way," as the *Upanishad* calls it), not to play the fairground entertainer.

Meditation in the penultimate stage should become gradually deeper
and deeper. At a certain moment the intellectual visions (that is
those emanating from the buddhi) fade away, and dhyana continues
"without support." What is meant here is clearly the strictly inde-
scribable state that the masters say is made up of silence and peace.
At this point a mutation occurs, and suddenly the yogi receives the
intuitive revelation of the unity of his atman with the universal atman
(brahman):

> *When he succeeds in practicing*
> *the meditation called "non-qualified,"*
> *the adept attains in twelve days*
> *that supreme goal of yoga*
> *called samadhi.*[5]

Now we have reached the final rung of yoga, the transcendent state to which the texts give the name samadhi. The word itself is a composite substantive containing the verb root *dha* (to place, to set down) and the verb prefixes *a* (indicating movement toward the subject speaking) and *sam* (fulfillment, perfection). What is conveyed, therefore, is a putting into place (*dha*) indicating a perfect (*sam*) interiorization (*a*). It has been translated in various ways: "enstasis," "seedless contemplation," "enstatic awareness without support," "perfect concentration," etc. The term "enstasis" (a neologism forged by the necessities of the occasion and used for the first time by Mircea Eliade) has the advantage of standing in clear opposition to the translation "ecstasy" which is found in a number of books but really will not do at all. Samadhi is in fact the exact opposite of ecstasy, for it is not "a going out of the being, a ravishment" but "a withdrawal back into the being, an interiorization," just as yoga is in no way a mystique but a psychosomatic method for achieving a return into one's self (and it must be borne in mind that the word "atman" is used in Sanskrit grammar as a reflective personal pronoun). The image of a saint being carried up from earth into heaven by the angels is at the opposite pole to that of the motionless yogi concentrating all the vital forces at his disposal, all the spiritual volence he has harnessed by using those forces, in an attempt to burst open the door that separates him from the Absolute. On the one hand we see passivity, self-abandonment, the action of grace, and on the other we see active striving pushed to its furthest limit, aggression, the feeling of owing everything to one's own efforts. From this point of view, the attempts some people have made to establish a "Christian yoga," or to assimilate yoga into Sufism, rest on fragile foundations. There are, indubitably, points of agreement at certain levels, possibilities for the adaptation of such practices, but the ideologies remain profoundly different, and opposed. The inexpiable hatred that has taken root over the past ten centuries between Hindus and Moslems arose in the first place from their theological differences: a visceral horror on the part of the monotheists for those pagans who claim to be able to become one with the Absolute, and a total inability on the part of the Hindus to tolerate the fanaticism of newcomers invoking their "one true faith" to forbid both polytheism and any attempt at spiritual identification.

Whatever the truth of this problem, it does not change the basic fact that samadhi is seen as the effective realization of the yoga program. Observation does show, however, that individuals who experience it "come down again" to the level of ordinary men, after longer or shorter periods of psychic "absence" that ought logically to be accompanied by actual physical "disappearance." In a word, the yogi ought to die when he realizes samadhi, since we are told that it consists in leaving the plane of existence:

> *When he has attained samadhi,*
> *when his individual soul*
> *has succeeded in uniting with the universal soul,*
> *the adept may, if he so wishes,*
> *abandon his body and take his rest*
> *forever in the breast of brahman,*
> *or, on the other hand, maintain*
> *his bodily integrity.*[6]

In practice, samadhi represents a radical transformation of the yogi as a human being. A sort of inner alchemy transmutes his body into a thing of radiance, just as his individual soul (jiva-atman) realizes its unity with the cosmic soul—in other words, with brahman:

> *When samadhi intervenes,*
> *the breath whirls in every direction*
> *like the molten gold*
> *in the alchemist's crucible:*
> *the body of flesh is transmuted at last*
> *into its divine form!*
> *Washed free of every stain,*
> *liberated from the numbed state*
> *in which its captive condition maintained it,*
> *the subtle body radiates splendor:*
> *behold it made of pure consciousness;*
> *it is the adept's very essence,*
> *since he is the universal soul*
> *present in all beings!*
> *This, they say, is the liberation*
> *that brings release from time and space!*[7]

This subtle transformation that makes the yogi's body radiant with splendor (invisible) in the state of samadhi is the sign of his victory over existence (that which the *Upanishad* just quoted calls "time and space"); the soul is henceforth authentically liberated, even though the individual continues to live. And it is for this reason that those yogis who have experienced samadhi and not died in doing so are called the "liberated-alive" (jivan-mukta).

Those who have reached this stage clearly live in a highly paradoxical fashion, since the very fact of living keeps them bound to the existential sphere to which their true selves nevertheless no longer truly belong. It is customary to say that they are no longer affected by any of the servitudes to which ordinary men are subjected: they do not suffer from cold or heat, no longer feel desire or regret, preserve a perfect equanimity in any circumstances, etc.[8] Moreover, they are naturally able to make use of all the various miraculous powers: live as long as they wish, employ their gifts of clairvoyance, ubiquity, invisibility, etc. Since they are now placed, by definition, "beyond good and evil," these supermen need no longer take any account of earthly values; everything is permitted to them. As one might expect, there are many yogis who, claiming (or sincerely believing) that they have attained samadhi, then take advantage of that attainment in order to "live in heaven" on earth. And metaphysically they are quite justified in doing so, insofar as their acts are all at once without cause and without effect. Without cause, because the jivan-mukta is by definition liberated from all desire (since all his vasanas have been destroyed); without effect because the liberated soul can on longer be affected by karman. Any act in such a situation must therefore be a gratuitous act, and this is why it is said of the jivan-mukta that he is in a state of absolute solitude (kaivalya). However, we must not deduce from this that others beings do not exist in relation to him, but on the contrary that he has left the sphere of existence and become identified with the One (atman/brahman). He is one where others are legion, and is no longer in any way affected by the universe to which he now belongs only in a fictive way.

The texts, of course, attempt to provide an account of the paradox constituted by the jivan-mukta's continuance in this world. If we ask how we are to understand that he is still alive, and that he still continues to act—sometimes in a scandalous manner—they answer by saying that his actions are directed to a higher end, one inaccessible to ordinary mortals. What appears aberrant or immoral to those ordinary mortals is in reality the external manifestation of a divine life unimaginable for the average man. Moreover, if the material, corporeal, psychic existence of the yogi continues, that is only because he has taken the decision to suspend the effects of the samadhi he has experienced. Wishing to avoid an irreversible situation that could result only in his actual departure from the world (in other words in his death), he has freely chosen (since to experience unity is also to experience true freedom) to remain on earth, in his body, in order to transmit his wisdom to those worthy of it through the process of initiation. Thus the jivan-mukta is transformed into a guru who journeys across India seeking for the disciples to whom he will be able to communicate his secret. When that task is accomplished, when the disciple has attained liberation in his turn, then the master provokes complete samadhi within himself and leaves life in a concrete sense. A yogi who dies is said to have "entered into samadhi," and to make it quite clear that this state transcends death, his body is not cremated (the obligatory form of body disposal among Hindus) but buried: it is as though the yogi were being placed "in storage" because no one knows whether this extended samadhi is or is not a true death. Often the master is even buried in the padma-asana or "lotus position" in token of the immortality attributed to him. The death of a jivan-mukta, then, is no more than a perpetual meditation for the benefit of his disciples, and the place of burial sometimes becomes a center of pilgrimage.[9]

To complete this account of yoga, however, it still remains for us to understand exactly what happens when the breath is held and the mind dissolves. The appearance of the miraculous powers and the inner alchemy that transfigures the yogi's body and spirit presuppose the existence of a subtle body within which these transformations can take place as well as that of a power capable of precipitating them. And instruction on the subject of the kundalini[10] and its operation—although strangely absent from Patanjali's *Yoga-Sutras* and from the *Bhagavad-Gita*—is in fact to be found in the *Upanishads* and above all in the *Tantras* (which gave their name to the branch of Hinduism known as Tantrism). It is to the presentation of this doctrine that the last part of this book will be devoted.

Part 4

The Eternal Feminine

10. The Divine Couple

hen Michelangelo painted God the Creator in all his majesty on the ceiling of the Sistine Chapel, he also painted a female figure seated close beside God. One might almost say pressed against him, did the Creator's sovereign mien and serenity of visage not forbid any such suggestion of familiarity between two personages that Christian theology is unable to link in such a way without the most extreme precaution. For this female figure very probably represents wisdom—the divine wisdom mentioned, it is true, in several passages of the Bible, but very rarely found personified like this. By painting "her" in this guise, Michelangelo was associating himself, perhaps unknowingly, with a current of thought that had manifested itself without interruption throughout our Middle Ages, one in which woman was promoted to the rank of inspiration and guide on the path of ritual progress (one thinks of Dante's Beatrice). The gnostic sects even went so far as to teach that the Holy Ghost was feminine in gender, so that their Trinity included a Father, a Son, and a Mother. But such concepts, having been declared heretical, had no place in the official theology of orthodox Christian churches, and found no more than furtive expression even in art or literature, as for instance in the *Divine Comedy,* or this representation of divine wisdom in the Sistine Chapel.

A Hindu, on the other hand, would find nothing astonishing about seeing Michelangelo's Wisdom seated next to God. He would recognize her as a goddess, the Lord's daughter or spouse. He would not only attribute to her the function of inspiration (or rather of inciting)[1] but would also say that the creation itself was in fact her work, while God remained impassive, inactive, in his role as sole witness of the unfurling of existential glamor. Going further, the Hindu would then explain that this glamor or magic (maya) is in fact nothing other than the goddess herself as she manifests herself in her cosmic form. Hearing him talk, you might receive the impression that only the female element plays any role in the process of cosmic development. If

you were to put this impression forward as an objection, however, the
Hindu would have no hesitation in dismissing it. God, he would say,
is merely a convenient word for denoting the Absolute (brahman),
and the Absolute, by definition, can never be qualified in any way;
consequently it cannot be the Creator, or the Father, or the Lord, or
the world could only come into being through the action of a goddess,
the Mother, the Sovereign Lady, who alone merits the name Creatress.
Such statements, I should quickly add, would probably not be accepted
by all Hindus (since there are many sects in which the male element is
believed to play an active role in the development of the cosmos), but
they do without doubt represent the beliefs of the great majority.

Indeed, during the past thousand years or so, worship of the goddess
in all her forms has come to occupy a dominant place in Hinduism.
Perhaps it did so even earlier, but no tangible evidence to support such
a claim has come down to us; whereas we do have texts dating from
about A.D. 1000 that establish the doctrine's foundations, set out the
ritual rules, and lay down its code of behavior. These texts have been
given the name of *Tantras* (books), which is why we speak of Tantrism
when referring to this branch of Hinduism. At other times the term
Shaktism is used to denote the same current of thought, because the
Sanskrit word *shakti* (power, force) is the one that best evokes the goddess's true nature: divine energy emanating from brahman, the concrete manifestation of her power of creation, etc. Whether called
Shaktism or Tantrism, however, the movement would not be truly
Hindu if it were not divided into many schools of thought, all engaged
in perpetual controversy with one another, and all remaining firmly in
agreement on essentials. Nor would it be truly Hindu if it had not
produced a multiplicity of goddesses, all with their place in a compli-
cated hierarchy (as in the case of the gods, genies, animal species, and
human castes), while at the same time agreeing that all of them together (and each in her individual way) represent the complex richness of the Eternal Feminine.

The amazing thing is that this ideology, so much alive still today
that Hindus look upon it as one of the essential forms of dharma,
could have remained for so long absent from India's sacred scriptures.
Neither the *Veda* nor the *Bhagavad-Gita* shows any awareness of it, or
at least ever alludes to it, even though it is impossible that it could
have appeared all at once, without cause and without history. Some

have suggested that it should be viewed as a resurgence of popular beliefs suppressed over a long period by the Brahmanic theologians, and it is indeed possible that the worship of female divinities at the village level could have played a part in the diffusion of the Tantric doctrines. But the doctrines themselves are far too erudite to owe their origin to any great extent to "tribal religions" (even if such religions could have subsisted in India after twenty centuries of Brahmanization).[2] In fact, the *Tantras* form a perfectly natural extension of the other revealed texts. They simply place their main emphasis on aspects of dharma that previous scriptural writings, for reasons of their own, had neglected. The *Bhagavad-Gita,* for example, being a dialogue between Vishnu—incarnated as Krishna—and Arjuna on the problem of how to act when faced with the difficult task of fulfilling the duties appropriate to one's status, cannot be expected to refer to doctrines outside those directly involved in its subject. In the same way, the *Veda,* because it is concerned almost exclusively with religious ritual, makes no more than glancing allusions to the individual cults and secret ceremonies that constitute the essence of Tantric practice. In both cases it would be mistaken to assume that these two works tells us everything about the religion of their time.

The same is true of the texts forming the foundation of yoga doctrine. As we saw earlier, the *Yoga-Sutras,* like the *Bhagavad-Gita,* makes absolutely no mention of the kundalini. The *Upanishads,* on the other hand, do give an important—and in some cases exclusive—place to expositions of the practices designed to awaken the kundalini, as well as to descriptions of its ascent through the subtle body. This contradiction, however, is only on the surface; here again we are dealing with specialized texts that should be taken as complementary to one another if we wish to arrive at a synthetic view of the *Yoga-Darshana.* The *Bhagavad-Gita* provides a metaphysical account of yoga and defines it in relation to dharma and religion (bhakti); the *Yoga-Sutras* provide technical instruction in yoga theory and practice, but their exposition of the ideas and facts on which these are based takes an extremely concise form and omits all detailed explanation (we saw earlier, for instance, that the definition of pratyahara is contained in a single sentence); the *Upanishads* fulfill the double function of inserting yoga into metaphysics while also providing secret, esoteric instruction concerned with the intrinsic reality of the things involved. Put another way, the *Bhagavad-Gita* says why one should practice yoga, the *Sutras* teach one how to do so, and the *Upanishads* reveal what actually happens as one advances along the path. Where the *Yoga-Sutras* content themselves with baldly stating that the eight stages will lead the individual to liberation, the *Upanishads* provide an account of the actual transformation process occurring within the yogi's personality. When Patanjali tells us that breath control, withdrawal of the senses, and meditation enable the individual who practices them to leave the sphere of existence, we can do no more than record his statement and cannot account for it on any but a logical level (which is what I have done in the previous chapters of this book). But by studying the *Upanishads* we can acquire the possibility of knowing "what lies behind" the *Sutras'* peremptory instructions. And "what lies behind" is in fact an entire theory of the subtle body, providing an account of the mysterious alchemy that induces the successive mutations of the human personality until it attains divine status and then, beyond even that achievement, realizes its definitive return to essence in a state of absolute isolation. It is to an exposition of this doctrine that the present and the following chapters will be devoted. I must warn the reader that I have made no attempt to give a total account of Tantrism, but only of those aspects of it that concern yoga.

Referring back to the schemes of the human composite (figures 1 and 2), we see that its structure is a clearcut dichotomy between those elements belonging to the realm of nature (prakriti) and those belonging to the realm of spirit (purusha). Thus the body, the sense organs, mental activity, and the intelligence form part of nature, while the atman alone is part of essence. This microcosmic classification is clearly analogous to that which orders the macrocosm: there too spirit is opposed to nature, essence to existence, purusha to prakriti. In formulating things in this way we remain on a strictly metaphysical plane that is accepted by all the great Hindu philosophical schools with only a few variations in vocabulary (the *Vedanta,* for instance, prefers to see maya[3] as the opposite of brahman) or doctrinal adjustments in line with their specific viewpoints. Tantrism, however, is not a darshana or "philosophic system" but a much broader synthesis embracing theory and practice, metaphysics and religion. It is a new or "modern" (in relation to the Vedic norm) expression of dharma as a whole. It cannot therefore remain on the level of pure speculation but transcends it by interpreting this dichotomy in religious terms (which do not replace the logical formulation but are superimposed upon it). For Tantrism too, purusha and prakriti are brahman and maya (spirit and nature, the Absolute and existential glamor), but they are above all the Lord-God and his creative-power (shakti). And the latter is no more abstract energy than the spirit is a pure metaphysical concept: she is a Goddess just as the spirit is God. In that lies Tantrism's originality; it is not merely a doctrine of opposition between Yin and Yang such as we find in Chinese tradition; nor is it a simple alchemy of wet and dry (to speak the language of our own Middle Ages). It is much more than that—a total interpretation of the universe, on all levels, including that of mythology.

On this latter level, God is given the name of Vishnu, or Shiva, or Krishna, etc.—according to the particular school—and the Goddess that of the particular god's traditional consort: Lakshmi, Parvati, Radha, etc. Or, if the "multiplicity" of nature is to be emphasized, as opposed to the essential oneness of the principle, then the shaktis too are multiplied. Mythologically this results, for example, in descriptions of Krishna surrounded by a swarm of *gopis* (cowgirls) all in love with him. I should add, however, that the Tantrism with which we are concerned here—in other words that form of it closest to yoga—is principally Shivaite and Vishnuite, and the *Yoga Upanishads* name the goddess either Lakshmi or Parvati (or substitutes for Parvati such as Durga, Uma, Kali).

Beyond these divergences between the various schools, however, the structure of the relations between God and Goddess(es) is every-where and always the same, identical in principle to that linking spirit and nature: on the one hand unique, immutable, absolute essence, on the other multiple, developing, relative existence. The relations es-tablished between them are those of husband and wife, the latter in Hindu tradition being the active partner, the one who expends energy in multiple activities in which the husband takes no hand (within the home, that is), while she is always defined entirely by her relation to him (she is neither wife nor mother except in relation to her hus-band). It will be remembered, for instance, that daughters do not receive the Brahmanic initiation (upanayana), and that this rite is re-placed in their case by marriage. Parvati or Lakshmi therefore exist only as emanations of Shiva or Vishnu, as manifestations of the latent powers that "slept" in the womb of purusha before the blossoming of creation. At the end of the cosmic cycle the goddesses (like the gods, genies, men, and all things) will be reabsorbed into the One, which will remain for a while in perfect balance before the evolutive process resumes its course with its first manifestation: the appearance of the Goddess-Nature who becomes responsible from that moment on for the organization of the cosmos.

Certain Tantric sects, consciously dualist in their theology, claim that prakriti cohabits with purusha eternally; at the end of the cosmic cycle "she" refurls the magic fabric of existence, reabsorbs into "herself" all its energies, and "falls asleep" beside the spirit until the moment comes for those elements and energies to be deployed again. More often, however, Tantric tradition prefers to subordinate the Goddess more clearly to her Lord and conceive of the end of the world as a return of the entire universe (i.e., all of nature) to its sole source the universal principle (purusha, or brahman, or atman), and since the Goddess is in fact indistinguishable from nature, she too cannot but be dissolved along with everything else into the undifferentiated Absolute. Yet the fact remains that substance itself, primal matter, cannot actually disappear, since Hinduism excludes creation ex nihilo. It must therefore subsist in some mysterious way within purusha as a virtuality that will be realized once more at the beginning of the new cycle. This presents a logical difficulty that the dualists overcome by positing the eternal continuance of both principles in time, side by side albeit closely interdependent. But it must be stressed again that Hinduism is profoundly opposed to dualism. It is in its entirety (above and beyond its passion for analysis and classification into minute subdivisions) a doctrine of the One. The quest for unity beyond the multiplicity of phenomena dominates all the methods of spiritual progress relating to dharma, so that from this point of view the dualist schools (which exist in India as they do elsewhere) are seen as heretical in nature.

Needless to say, the situation just described on the level of the "great creation" is to be found reflected feature by feature in the microcosm of the human being, in accordance with the principle of analogy upon which, as we have seen, the entire edifice of Hindu philosophy is built. Within us, therefore, since we exist, the male and female principles must likewise cohabit. The former is purusha, present in us as it is in any fragment of the universe, no matter how small; the latter is clearly prakriti, at work in us as it is everywhere else in order that the being we are shall be born, develop, subsist a while, then die in accordance with the common norm. For terminological convenience the first is called atman (a masculine word in Sanskrit) and the second kundalini. As far as the atman is concerned, it is hardly necessary to repeat here what has been said on so many occasions in previous chapters. I will merely remind the reader that it possesses all the characteristics of purusha (oneness, essentiality, impassibility, etc.) since it *is* purusha (or brahman, whichever you wish to call it). It will be remembered that, although immutable and "without qualities," atman (and therefore brahman/purusha) is knowing, so that it is also said to be sach-chid-ananda (being-consciousness-joy). We must therefore remember that liberation, deliverance from existence by returning to the Absolute, is not an annihilation but, on the contrary, an advance, a transition upward to the sphere of essence, in which all is perfection: perfection of being (finally unshackled from the limitations of existence), perfection of consciousness (in which consciousness has become pure concentration on itself), perfection of joy (in which consciousness has become pure and eternal joy as opposed to the universe of suffering constituted by the natural world). It is this notion of cosmic consciousness that makes it possible to explain how relations can exist between the Absolute and the Relative, between spirit and nature, between atman and kundalini.

In other words, the kundalini is shakti, the divine power incarnated in our body and inextricably involved in its destiny. In order to convey precisely what this power is, the tradition employs various symbols. One of them is that of fire. In ordinary men this fire is no more than a few smoldering embers providing just sufficient power to maintain the organism's normal functions from birth to death. But potentially it is a tremendous source of energy, the same energy that moves the whole universe, causes the sun to shine, makes possible the existence of thousands of millions of living beings, etc. Most of us do not even know of its existence, and are therefore totally unable to harness it in any way, but the initiate, guided by his guru, learns to recognize (to "see") this fire and eventually, by following the stages of yoga, succeeds in fanning the sleeping flames to life. Suddenly it roars up into a vast conflagration that sets the yogi totally aflame until it has burned away within him every barrier to spiritual progress. Then, this conflagration over, the fully "realized" shakti is reabsorbed into the atman. And that is liberation, moksha, the sole aim of all yoga teaching.

The other symbol, more often given primacy (although it is always used in conjunction with that of fire), represents the shakti as a woman-serpent slumbering inside the individual's body. It is said that there exists a cavity (cave, nest) at the base of the trunk in which the serpent lies coiled around upon itself, its head biting its tail (hence the name kundalini, which means "she who is curled around upon herself"). Usually, in the ordinary individual, the serpent gives off just enough energy to maintain life, but when the yogi succeeds in awakening her, she rears up, hissing like a cobra stirred up by the snake charmer's stick or awakened by her master's flute, and gradually makes her way up inside the body until she reaches the head, where she opens a hole (called *brahmarandhra*: "the hole of brahman," or *brahmadvara*: "the door of brahman") through which the atman can escape, just like a bird when the door of its cage has been opened.

This process of the kundalini's awakening, her ascent, then her emergence at the moment when the yogi reaches his goal, will be explained in detail later. For the moment it is enough to stress the fact that the yogi, by his use of yoga, forces the shakti to behave in a way contrary to the natural course of its existence. Indeed, one might even go so far as to say that the shakti ought to rebel against an enterprise that is aimed at nothing less than her own destruction. For the goal being sought is the total isolation (kaivalya) of the atman when it absorbs the yogi's divine energy into itself, thereby causing it literally to cease existing, since liberation is the dissolution (*laya*) of everything within the human structure that is not the atman itself. The texts do in fact stress the difficulty of the undertaking due to the "natural" (i.e., deriving from the shakti) resistance of the body and the thought organ motivated by their instinct for self-preservation, etc. But they also add, in the same breath as it were, that the shakti collaborates in her own destruction because she is a goddess and on that account aspires to union with her husband: she feels a desire to approach him more closely, to unite with him, to melt into him, even at the price of her life.

At a yet deeper level, Tantrism, like yoga, is a *sadhana* (method of spiritual realization) that uses nature to annihilate nature, the body to tame the body, thought to dissolve thought, and so on. Here again we find something that recalls the alchemical tradition in which the lead must be destroyed in order for the gold to appear: every transmutation is the annihilation of a form in order that the element may reveal itself in its original, nonformed purity. But whether it be in the work of the alchemist or in the practice of yoga, it is violence that is at work, in the form of a will to dominate the universe: the yogi, like the alchemist, looks upon the natural world both as an adversary (since it constitutes a screen between him and the Absolute) and as an ally (since it is by making use of nature that he will succeed in conquering it). Ramakrishna, known as an ardent worshiper of Kali, said that the love he bore for her was a danger to his spiritual progress. At one point he allowed it to become an indulgence, and the delight with which her worship filled his life became a major obstacle by making him forget the goal he had set himself. He was therefore obliged to smash, to tear asunder the image of the goddess in order to reach the Absolute. Only afterward did he realize that it was Kali herself who had given him the strength, the courage to accomplish this apparently sacrilegious act. Such attitudes are constantly honored in the Tantric texts, which stress again and again the idea that it is by using evil that one triumphs over evil (and we know that certain Tantric practices, condemned as shockingly immoral, are aimed solely at enabling the adept to make use of the energy required for their realization in order to destroy desire within himself root and branch).

Before going any further it would be as well to emphasize that the male-female symbolism is very concrete in the Tantric tradition. Even though it is true that its ultimate expression is the union of spirit with nature, the fact still remains that the word used to denote spirit is purusha, a term whose primary meaning as early as the Vedic period was "the male." And that is why the symbol that best represents it is that of the *linga* (erect phallus), while prakriti is represented by the *yoni* (womb, uterus). Throughout India we find representations of the universe in the form of a cylindrical stone standing on a triangular plinth: the image of a linga rising from a womb. The ubiquity of these representations, the worship accorded them, and the veneration in which they are held are proof of the immense influence Tantrism has had on the Indian mind for many centuries. But the most important point here for us is that in this form the union of the two principles seems to give purusha an active role, which would be in direct contradiction of all that we have said so far about its impassibility. One may take, for example, the most ancient of the cosmogonies, found in the *Rig-Veda,* that depict the birth of the world as a marriage between heaven and earth in which the feminine element is pure passivity and the masculine element active power (the symbolism being that of the plowman opening up the belly of the earth with his plowshare in order to implant his seed in it). But perhaps this Vedic symbolism applies solely to the moment of the primal impulse, envisaged in its most concrete form, and is not intended to refer to the consequences that will ensue once the initial fertilization is over and the earth must begin to feed the embryo in its (her) womb before bringing it into the world (all living creatures are looked upon as daughters of the earth from the Vedic point of view). As for Tantrism, it teaches that purusha is at the same time the linga and the seed, both eternally present and available. At the moment when the evolutive process is triggered, the drop of sperm finds itself miraculously localized in a womb which is also eternally present and available. From that point onward all the labor of gestation, delivery, suckling, rearing, and so on will be the exclusive work of the mother, while the father contents himself with the role of passive witness of his wife's activity and his child's development. There are numerous mythological legends that include a Parvati infuriated by the apparent indifference of her husband Shiva, who sits motionless on top of Mount Kailasa, meditating, while she is obliged to take care of the household and their son's upbringing. Others tell how the god flies into a rage because the child has disturbed him in his yoga exercises, and so on. These are naive but significant expressions of the fundamental doctrine concerning the relations between nature and spirit, and it is the way in which these relations manifest themselves, concretely, during the prescribed yoga exercises, that we must now investigate.

11. The Subtle Body

In order to understand the mechanism by which yoga exercises succeed in awakening the divine power, we must first understand what those who practice them mean by "the subtle body" (*sukshma-sharira*). The idea behind it is that the corporeal constituent making up one quarter of the human composite (the other three quarters being thought, intelligence, and soul) is itself formed of two complex and superimposed structures; one is the material mass formed by the skeleton, the muscles, the viscera, the organs of perception and action, while the other is a sort of invisible mandala formed by a combination of symbolic (but also very real) geometric figures. The body proper, the one accessible to our senses, is referred to as the "gross" body (*sthula*). This is the body whose anatomy had very early on been explored and precisely codified by doctors—by which of course I mean physicians—skilled in the ancient Indian medical tradition, which in many respects resembled that of Hippocrates. Vedic religion, in which animal sacrifices were obligatory, had assisted in developing an exact knowledge of the internal physical structure of animals and men (for human victims were occasionally sacrificed too), since its rituals entailed subsequent dismemberment of the corpses and examination of the internal organs, a practice very similar to that found in Rome, Greece, Carthage, and indeed everywhere that this type of liturgy existed. Which means that the Indians were perfectly well aware of the purposes served by the muscles, the stomach, etc. Nor were they ignorant of the fact that mental activity was centered in the brain. And having observed the causal links between different kinds of wounds and the disabilities they produced, they also understood the importance of breathing and digestion to life. They were therefore in no danger of confusing the circulation of the blood with that of air in the body, or of believing that the heart was the organ of thought, a fact important to bear in mind if one is to arrive at a correct evaluation of what is said about the subtle body.

As far as yoga is concerned, there is another body, no less real for being inaccessible to the senses, coexisting with the one we all know. The epithet "subtle" that is applied to it comes from the vocabulary of alchemy; it indicates both invisibility and superiority, because it goes without saying that the subtle body is more important than the gross body insofar as it is in fact "beyond the senses." Here again we are dealing with the principle of analogy so fundamental to Hindu thought, as we have already seen in many other domains in the course of this book. The gross body is in fact an analogue of the subtle body, by which is meant that the latter is the model from which the gross body is derived, even though the reproduction (the gross body) must of necessity be inferior in quality to the original (the subtle body). We shall thus find in the subtle body all the properties present in the gross body, but magnified, multiplied to their maximum power.

It is even claimed that if our organs succeed in functioning, if the gross body is able to exist and to subsist at all, it is only because it is directed, "informed"[1] by the subtle body. Not that the latter is conceived of as a conscious, active persona; the subtle body, I repeat, is a structure of reference, an image, a yantra. But the fact is that nothing can exist in the universe without a higher model. The Bible tells us that man is only as he is because he was created "in God's image," and the Hindus would find no difficulty in subscribing to that statement, except that they would always tend to prefer a multiplicity of models and copies. In short, the Hindu tradition believes in the existence of molds from which the tangible forms that make up the universe accessible to empirical knowledge are reproduced in vast quantities. The beauty of the world in which we live is as nothing compared to that of these innumerable archetypes that combine to form the vast mandala of the cosmic wheel continually turning from beginning to end of the cycle.

It should be added that the differences between men, the greater or lesser imperfection of their gross bodies, are due to the vasanas accumulated by them during their successive existences in accordance with the law of karman, while the human model (the subtle body) is, in contrast, unique, identical in all men, without imperfections; it knows no mutations but remains unchanged until the end of time. The frequency of the "pressings," their multiplicity, and their defects, can all be inputed to the clumsiness of the humans responsible (while under the sway of desire), not to the model nor, needless to say, to the author of the model (nature, prakriti).

It should be stressed that this principle of analogy operates on many levels: just as the gross body is analogous to the subtle body, so the latter in its turn is analogous to the universe. We must understand clearly that the subtle body is the perfect microcosm (of which the gross body is an imperfect representation), but that this microcosm is in its turn made in the image of the macrocosm. We ought therefore to find in the human body (subtle and gross) the selfsame elements that constitute the universe, not only earth, water, fire, etc., but also the stars, the sun, the planets, and even its rivers, seas, etc. One yoga text eloquently expresses precisely this notion:

> *In your body is Mount Meru*
> *encircled by the seven continents;*
> *the rivers are there too,*
> *the seas, the mountains, the plains,*
> *and the gods of the fields.*[2]
> *Prophets are to be seen in it, monks,*[3]
> *places of pilgrimage*
> *and the deities presiding over them.*
> *The stars are there, and the planets,*
> *and the sun together with the moon;*
> *there too are the two cosmic forces:*
> *that which destroys, that which creates;*
> *and all the elements: ether,*
> *air and fire, water and earth.*
> *Yes, in your body are all things*
> *that exist in the three worlds,*
> *all performing their prescribed functions*
> *around Mount Meru;*
> *he alone who knows this*
> *is held to be a true yogi.*[4]

The matter could hardly be put with greater clarity. We shall see later that each of these cosmic components has its precise place in the mandala and, in consequence, in some particular part of the gross body. So when we read, for example, that "the sun, the moon, and fire are present in man's heart," we are to understand by this that the organ in question is situated within the gross body in that place where, in the subtle body, one finds the "center" corresponding to the position of those celestial bodies in the cosmic wheel.

Another example: according to Indian tradition the earth has seven continents (regarded as islands) arranged around a mountain named Meru whose summit is the home of the gods (and thus similar to the Greeks' Olympus). This arrangement is similar to that of the universe as a whole (which gravitates around an axis: brahman the cosmic axle), while the earth in its turn is the model for the structure of the subtle body, in which we shall find a central pillar with seven centers organized around it, analogous to the seven continents. And finally there comes the gross body modeled upon the image of the subtle body, so that the spine can be seen as an analogue of Mount Meru, the cosmic support, brahman, and so on.

So we have a whole hierarchy (gross body in the image of the subtle body, which reproduces the schema of the world we live in, which is in its turn an analogue of the total universe) that is capable of even further diversification, since naturally the intermediary world (that of the genies and angels) is analogous to heaven (home of the gods), etc. But let us not linger over the details; what concerns us here is the idea that the subtle body is made in the image of the universe and that the powers of nature are all present within it. I hardly need add that if yoga works, it does so by revealing the existence of the subtle body and enabling the practitioner to employ its latent energies.

To begin with, viewed very broadly, the subtle body is divided into five main sections, arranged in an appropriate hierarchy, and each related to one of the cosmic elements. One of the *Yoga Upanishads* provides a detailed account of these divisions and indicates how the yogi can gain mastery over each of the elements by meditating on the deity that governs them:

> *In the adept's body*
> *the section between feet and knees*
> *belongs to the element earth;*
> *the earth is square,*
> *it is yellow,*
> *it is symbolized*
> *by the syllable* lam.

The yogi causes the vital breath to enter
this part of his body
by sounding lam *within it.*
Then he meditates on Brahma,
the golden colored god,
with four arms, and four faces,
while holding his breath in,
for five times twenty-four measures,
and by this means makes himself master
of the earthly element
and protects himself from death.[5]

The procedure is clear: the yogi is first brought to an awareness of the existence of the element earth within him and a knowledge of its location; then, by employing pranayama (breath control), he suspends his breathing for a considerable period (a little over three minutes), and directs his breath down to that part of his body belonging to earth; at this point he acquires an intuitive knowledge of that element and sees that in the mandala of his body it is a yellow square with the syllable *lam* inscribed within it. Then he must try to make that syllable sound there, and if he succeeds he receives a revelation of the deity who presides over the element of earth (the creator-god Brahma), and by meditating on that deity he acquires mastery over the cosmic force symbolized by earth, the yellow square, and the god Brahma, so that henceforth he has nothing more to fear from it.

And so with all the other elements. In ascending order, we find water (between knees and anus), fire (between anus and heart), air (between heart and eyebrows), and lastly ether (between the eyebrows and the top of the head). The geometric shapes are a crescent for water, a triangle for fire, a hexagon for air, a circle for ether. The syllables are, respectively, *vam, ram, yam, ham,* and the deities, Vishnu, Rudra, Ishvara, Shiva.[6] The mastery acquired over each of the elements, together with the consequent protection of the major gods, enables the yogi not only to dismiss all further fear of perishing on earth, in water, or in fire, but also to fly through the air and even travel through cosmic space! So now it is quite clear how the "miraculous powers" are in fact the realization (siddhi) of virtualities we all carry within us but which the practice of meditation alone—when carried out in accordance with the rules of yoga—can reveal to us. We must remember that, in the Hindu tradition, to know something is to take possession of it, to become united with it (just as in biblical terms "to know" a woman means to possess her sexually).

TABLE 1   THE FIVE ELEMENTS OF THE SUBTLE BODY

Location	Element	Shape	Syllable	Deity	Benefit
between feet and knees	earth	yellow square	*lam*	Brahma	victory over earthly death
between knees and anus	water	white crescent	*vam*	Vishnu	no risk of death by water
between anus and heart	fire	red triangle	*ram*	Rudra	no risk of death by fire
between heart and eyebrows	air	black hexagon	*yam*	Ishvara	power to move like the wind through the air
between eyebrows and top of the head	ether	blue circle	*ham*	Shiva	power to journey through cosmic space

The meditation that makes possible the realization of the elemental powers is accompanied, as we have just seen, by a retention of the breath. This is something we are already quite familiar with, since we have seen in previous chapters that this retention is necessary to produce sense withdrawal (pratyahara) and to enable attention (dharana) to be concentrated into a single point. But here we learn something new: the breath must be guided, inside the body, toward some specific area—feet, belly, heart, eyebrows, and so on. Clearly this can only be understood with reference to the subtle body, since the Hindus know just as well as we do that "material" air penetrates no further than the lungs. Yet this internal circulation is of the very highest importance since it is what determines the success or otherwise of the meditation. The texts are categorical on this point: it is only when the inhaled and held breath has reached the selected area that the yogi acquires the intuitive knowledge of the power (or deity) that he wishes to use for his spiritual progress. We are now at the heart of the yoga doctrine: if everything is directed toward the practice of pranayama (breath control), it is because the breath (prana) is the motive force of spiritual progress, the catalyst that triggers the alchemical process by which the profane aspirant is transmuted into a true yogi, one who has "seen" the latent powers and therefore realized them within himself.

This inner circulation of the breath is made possible by the existence of an intricate network of channels which form a kind of web that is the structure of the subtle body. These channels are clearly analogous to the veins and arteries of the gross body but must in no way be confused with them. I repeat, Indian medicine was well aware, twenty-five centuries ago, that the air we inhale fills our lungs and not our livers or our brains. The Sanskrit name for these channels running through the subtle body is *nadis,* a technical term (also used in medicine) that sounds like the word for rivers—also *nadis* (the only difference between the two words lying in the phonetic nature of the *d*). Yoga texts love to play on this ambiguity. Thus, for example, the author of the passage from the *Shiva-Samhita* quoted above, when speaking symbolically of Mount Meru and the rivers flowing down from it, is really referring to the axis of the subtle body and to the channels that run through it.

These nadis are so numerous that it is impossible to count them. To express this infinity, the texts give figures running into hundreds of thousands (in the *Shiva-Samhita,* 2.13, for instance, the number is 350,000), but they all agree in adding that only a few of them have any importance from the point of view of yoga. It would seem, in practice, that the primary function of these innumerable channels is to constitute the ideal model upon which the gross body is to be constructed at the moment of conception. So that there ought in fact to be as many nadis in the subtle body as there are veins, arteries, nerves, capillaries, etc., in the gross body.

The yogi, however, needs no more than a dozen of these nadis to effect the circulation of breath through his body toward the areas that concern him. To return to the example of meditation on the element earth, for instance, he must find the path through his subtle body that will lead the prana (breath) down to his feet. To do so he must visualize the inner mandala and then find his way through the labyrinth of nadis, an operation recognizable as the archetypal initiation test, and we know that labyrinth symbolism is common to all ancient traditions. The most important operation of all, however, is the awakening of the kundalini, which, as we explained earlier, resides in a cave situated in the lowest part of the trunk. The yogi must therefore discover those nadis which irrigate that area of the subtle body. And when he has familiarized himself with the whole complex network and its hundreds of thousands of channels, he will find that three of them only are concerned with that region of the body.

These three nadis are called the sushumna, the ida, and the pingala. One of them, the sushumna, is central, while the other two are situated on either side of it. The image formed is identical with that of the caduceus carried by Hermes/Mercury: a straight wand with two snakes coiled around it. More specifically, the three nadis meet in the cave where the snake-kundalini is coiled; their sources are in the head (ida and pingala at the level of the nose, sushumna at the top of the skull); the outer two cross the sushumna, and each other, four times as they wind downward, while the sushumna remains straight and rigid like the wand of the caduceus or the world axis. The intersections are situated at points on a vertical axis corresponding to the locations of certain parts of the gross body (see figure 9). But, as we now know, the word "heart," say, in this context does not refer in any way to the anatomical heart, but rather to a center in the subtle body (to a point in the inner mandala) analogically situated at the same "latitude" as the heart. As we shall see later, these centers play an all-important role in the yogi's spiritual progress. Each of these three principal nadis is the ideal expression of a complex symbolism that helps us to understand the role attributed to them in the technique employed for awakening the kundalini and inducing it to ascend upward inside the subtle body until liberation is attained. When the specific function of the nadis (that of conducting the vital breath through the body) is being stressed, it is explained that the pingala and the ida have their sources "at the level of the nose." The ida is said to start in the left nostril, the pingala in the right, and the inhaled air is said to travel down through the ida as far as the base of the trunk then make its way up again via the pingala in order to be exhaled through the right nostril. Though in fact, the choice of one of these nadis in particular for either the upward or downward channel cannot be of any importance since we find the texts contradicting one another on this point; the *Dhyanabindu Upanishad* instructs the yogi to "draw in the air

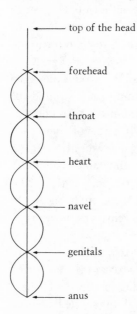

Fig. 9
Channels of the subtle
body: their intersections

Labels on figure: top of the head, forehead, throat, heart, navel, genitals, anus

through the left nostril" (1.20), while the *Yogakundalini Upanishad* says (1.24) that "the outside air should be inhaled through the right nostril alone," only to add three lines later that "the air should be inhaled through both nostrils and carried gently through both left and right canals." All we need to remember, then, is that the two outer nadis serve as paths for the breath and that they are employed in various ways by different schools. Moreover, the texts frequently prefer to avoid superimposing the pattern of the three nadis on that of the anatomical breathing channels (those in the nose, that is) and therefore invert the image by saying that the three nadis have their common source at the base of the trunk, in the kundalini's cave. In which case the head becomes destination rather than source: the ida and the pingala intersect for a sixth and final time at the latitude of the forehead ("between the eyebrows"), while the sushumna alone continues on higher, up to the top of the skull (and even further according to some traditions).

The ida, because it is to the left, lies in the realm of feminine symbolism: it is the moon and presents an aquatic (wet) and cold character; the pingala, on the right, has the masculine qualities of dryness and heat and is the sun. As for the sushumna, it transcends both these pairs of opposites; it is neither male nor female but both at the same time (one might say "neuter" if the term is understood to have a

TABLE 2   THE THREE CHANNELS OF THE SUBTLE BODY

Name	Location	River	Color	Heavenly Body	Symbolism
ida	left	Ganges	pale yellow	moon	female
pingala	right	Yamuna	red	sun	male
sushumna	center	Sarasvati	diamond	fire	"neuter"

positive value); it is the fire whose light the Hindus think of as "primal" (the sun being no more than an "incarnation," as it were, of this universal fire). The respective colors associated with the three are pale yellow for ida, red for pingala, the transparency ("the color of diamond") for sushumna. Lastly, there is a geographical symbolism: the ida is the Ganges (the word *ganga* is feminine in Sanskrit), the pingala is the Yamuna (modern Jumna, a tributary of the Ganges flowing in from the right), and the sushumna is the Sarasvati. It is important to know, in this context, that the confluence of these three

rivers is regarded as one of the most sacred places in India. Near the
city that the Moslems called Allahabad (its official name in modern
India), the waters of the Yamuna can indeed be seen mingling with
those of the Ganges, but you would seek in vain for a view of the
Sarasvati: that river (today called the Sutlej) is a tributary not of the
Ganges but of the Indus. But Hindus believe that the Sarasvati flows
into the confluence of the Ganges and Yamuna subterraneanly (or in
some invisible way) and becomes married to them. And the mystery
that surrounds this marriage means that the Sarasvati is looked upon
as the holiest of all rivers in the world (that is, in the "subtle" universe, inaccessible to our senses).

Moreover, the symbolism involved is much more complex than the
broad lines already given might suggest. Looked at from another
standpoint, it can actually be inverted: certain *Tantras,* for example,
teach that the male seed is an attribute of the ida (which is quite
normal, since the moon in Hindu symbolism is a male character associated with Shiva and presiding over masculine sexual activity), in
which case the pingala is seen as being associated with the phenomenon
of ovulation (because menstrual blood is red and symbolizes the sun).
But ultimately these variations are of no great importance, since the
essential thing for yoga is to reach the confluence of the three rivers
(and in the case of the symbolism just mentioned this meeting of the
three rivers will take the form of a marriage analogous to that between
Shiva and Parvati). Other accounts say that the sushumna is not single
but made up in its turn of three separate elements. These are usually
represented as being in the form of two concentric sheaths enclosing
the third element called *chitra* (the shining); but this symbolism
(which is a further application of the analogy principle, the sushumna
itself being the image of its own association with the ida and the
pingala!) plays no more than a very secondary role in descriptions of
the kundalini's ascent, so that we can ignore it here.

The important thing for us remains the essential function performed
by the nadis, which is that of conveying the breath through the body.
The following passage from the *Yogatattva Upanishad* (1.36) clearly
sets out the technique the yogi is to use:

> *Holding his body very straight,*
> *the yogi will first salute*
> *his chosen deity;*

then he will stop up with his thumb
the right nostril where the pingala has its source
so as to inhale air gently
through the left nostril where the ida has its source.
Then he will hold in his breath
as long as is possible,
then expel it gradually,
without forcing, through the left nostril.
Later, he will inhale again,
through the left nostril this time,
conveying the air down into his belly
which he will gradually fill.
After having kept it there
as long as he can,
he will expel it through his right nostril,
gently, without forcing.
He will continue in this way,
inhaling through one nostril,
afterwards exhaling through the other,
each time holding the breath
as long as he can.

Apart from showing that the yogi must employ the two channels alternately (which is tantamount to saying that they do not have separate specialized functions), this passage makes it quite clear that breathing envisaged in this way (with the breath being conveyed to a given area of the body via the nadis) constitutes an alchemical operation leading to a transformation of the practitioner's body. When this has been achieved, it remains for him to awaken the kundalini and cause her to ascend through the central nadi to the top of his head. It is this final operation that we must now look into.

12. The Power of the Serpent

he yogi who has attained complete mastery over the technique of breathing, and who has been able by this means to isolate himself totally from the external world, succeeds in "seeing" the interior of his body or, in other words acquires intuitive knowledge of the secret mandala that his subtle body forms. Having unraveled the tangled web of the nadis, he reaches the end of his journey of initiation and penetrates to the most inward part of himself, at the base of the trunk, where there is a cave located at the foot of the cosmic mountain. In this cave the yogi perceives three things: a fire of glowing embers, a sleeping serpent, and the threefold orifice of the three principal channels, the ida, the pingala, and the sushumna:

> *The divine power,*
> *the kundalini, shines*
> *like the stem of a young lotus;*
> *like a snake, coiled around upon herself,*
> *she holds her tail in her mouth*
> *and lies resting half asleep*
> *at the base of the body.*[1]

The great task now is to awaken this serpent, which means, in symbolic trems, to achieve conscious awareness of the presence within us of shakti or "cosmic power" and begin to use it in the service of spiritual progress.

To succeed in this task the yogi will need to summon up all the strength he has at his command since yoga has enabled him to reach the stage at which he can practice dhyana (transcendental meditation). Taking up the yoga position he has personally found most suitable (usually the siddha-asana or "position of perfection" described in chapter 7), he closes the windows of his body one by one (in other words achieves pratyahara or "sense withdrawal" and concentrates all his attention on a single point (dharana). At this point his mental activity is totally suspended, and the buddhi (intelligence), reflecting the light of the atman, takes over. Illuminated in this way, the yogi's supraconscious will (i.e., the intellectual vitality of the buddhi as opposed to the manas, which has been "dissolved" by dharana) is directed upon the breath inhaled and retained in pranayama. Guided in this way, the breath (prana) is conveyed down to the base of the trunk and introduced via either the ida or the pingala into the cave where the kundalini lies coiled.

The entry of the prana produces an abrupt animation of the fire in the cave: the embers blossom into flame and the god Agni (Fire) brightens into splendor. The heat, the brightness, and the roar of the now flaming fire combine to waken the serpent at least from its torpor.

> *The yogi conveys the prana*
> *down into the muladhara;*
> *the air thus drawn in awakens*
> *the fire-below that lay sleeping.*
> *Meditating on the pranava*
> *that is brahman,*
> *concentrating his thought,*
> *he causes the breath to rise*
> *mingled with the fire-below*
> *as far as the navel and beyond*
> *within the subtle body.*[2]

It is clear from this text that the process of awakening the kundalini is in the first place a result of meditation (dhyana); it is because he is meditating on pranava (that is, brahman represented by the sound *om*) that the yogi succeeds in fanning the fire-below into flame. And we should note that the *Upanishad* also instructs the yogi that he must cause the breath, once vivified by the fire-below, to rise up inside his subtle body. The idea here is that the kundalini is assisted by the prana and the god Agni: having awakened her they continue to accompany her in her gradual ascent.

The other interesting point brought out by this quotation is the mention of the first center of the subtle body, the *muladhara*. And it is now time in fact to explain that the internal mandala—consisting,

as we have seen, of a vast number of nadis (rivers, channels) forming a complex network— also comprises a series of geometrical figures,
seven in number, spaced out along a vertical axis running from the
base of the trunk up to the top of the head. These figures are usually
called chakras, a Sanskrit word that has the primary meaning of
"wheel" (of a chariot) but can be used more broadly to denote any
circular object, such as a disk, a potter's wheel, a cyclic period, and
so on. The universe itself, for instance, is an immense chakra (the
cosmic wheel) that revolves eternally around a hub (brahman). All
the chakras within the subtle body are therefore primarily circles, whatever other geometrical figures they may have inscribed within those
circles. Moreover, these centers are also referred to as lotuses (*padma*),
but it must be remembered that all stylized representations of the lotus
in Indian iconography are based on the circle (surrounded by a vari-
able number of petals), except of course when the flower has not yet
opened (the lotus bud, often used as a symbol of virtuality awaiting
realization). In fact this iconographic stylization is often taken so far
that one is unsure whether to recognize certain figures as a wheel or
as a lotus. The average Indian is not at all sure whether the symbol
that appears on his national flag is a lotus or a wheel, and from his
point of view it does not matter much, since the symbolism is the
same: that circular structure with its radiating beams is beyond doubt
an image of dharma.

Obviously the seven chakras are precisely located within the subtle
body, and by analogy with the gross body they are said to be situated
at the same height as such and such an organ. But I must emphasize yet
again that the chakras must not be thought of as coincident with any
part of the gross body; they are superimposed images indicating the
confluent points of particular vital forces, the activity of which sets
the forces of the gross body in motion, but which remain substantially
distinct from them (they subsist after death and contribute to the
animation of the fetus at the moment of reincarnation in another body,
in accordance with the laws of transmigration). It is therefore more
correct to say that the seven chakras are situated "at the same latitude"
as certain parts of the body, as we said in the previous chapter when
referring to the presence of the cosmic elements within the inner mandala. With this proviso in mind we can say that the first chakra is level
with the anus; the second with the genitals; the third with the navel; the
fourth with the heart; the fifth with the throat; the sixth with the

forehead; the seventh with the top of the head. Here are a few more details about each one individually:

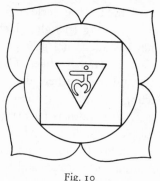

Fig. 10
The muladhara

1. The first chakra is called the *muladhara,* because it is situated at the base (*mula,* "root") of the trunk (see figure 10). Its geometrical representation is a circle containing a square and a downward pointing triangle.[3] Viewed as a lotus, the muladhara has four petals; its dominant color is yellow, and the related mantra is the syllable *lam.* As the presence of the square and the color yellow indicate, the symbolism here is that of the element earth, further stressed by the downward pointing triangle (image of the yoni, the female sexual organ). It is sometimes said that the yogi should perceive a linga in the center of the yoni, which is a way of making him understand that the male and female principles coexist in all living beings.

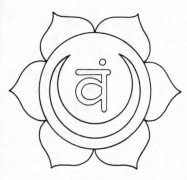

Fig. 11
The svadhishthana

2. The second chakra is located at the level of the sexual organs and is called the *svadhishthana,* which implies that it is the site of whatever constitutes the individual's specific personality (see figure 11). The geometrical representation is a circle containing a crescent moon. As a lotus, this center has six petals; its color is white; its mantra is the syllable *vam.* Here we recognize the sexual symbolism that is bound up in Hinduism with the moon and the color white: the moon god, it is said, travels through the world during the nights when he is new and fertilizes the waters, which then give birth to the plants that will serve in their turn as food for beasts and men, and so on. The moon god is always present when two living beings unite: it is he who deposits the drop of sperm in the womb. The cosmic element of this chakra is therefore water.

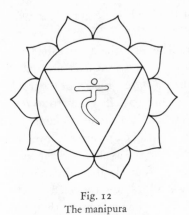

Fig. 12
The manipura

3. The third chakra, called the *manipura,* is located on the latitude of the navel (see figure 12). It is represented by a circle enclosing a downward pointing triangle which sometimes has additional geometric protuberances (rather like *T*'s) which are said to be either "doors" for effecting entrance into the diagram or stylized svastikas (the svastika or auspicious sign is a symbol of fire). As a lotus, the manipura has ten petals; its color is red, and the appropriate mantra is the syllable *ram.* The symbolism here is that of fire, as indicated by the color red and possibly by the protuberances sometimes added to the triangle, if it is true that they are svastikas. The presence of fire in this region of the body is explained by the fact that Hindu tradition views digestion as the destruction of food by an inner fire, a process of combustion that reduces the food to ashes (feces) while fortifying our vital energy (thought of as a warm, luminous flame).

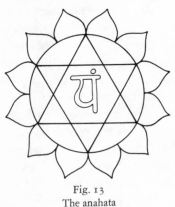

Fig. 13
The anahata

4. The fourth chakra is called the *anahata* (see figure 13). It is located at the level of the heart, and its circle is occupied by two superimposed triangles, one pointing up and one down, forming a six-pointed star like Solomon's seal. As a lotus, this center has twelve petals; its color is gray; its mantra is *yam;* and its cosmic element is air. The symbolism here is complex; the two triangles indicate the ultimate union and fulfillment of the male principle (upward-pointing triangle) and the female (downward-pointing triangle), so that here they have a cosmic, universal value, whereas that of the linga within the yoni seen in the muladhara was restricted to that of specifically sexual union. The other aspect of the fourth chakra's symbolism concerns the element air. Here it is not air as "vital breath" but air as

atmosphere and the conveyer of sound that is involved. The name of the chakra in fact implies that it emits a mysterious sound comparable to that which would be produced by an un- (*an-*) -beaten (*-ahata*) drum, which is another way of saying that the sound in question lies outside the categories of the world of the senses. And as the texts indicate, the sound that reverberates within the lotus of the heart is *om,* brahman as sonic vibration.[4]

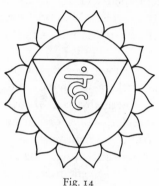

Fig. 14
The vishuddha

5. The fifth chakra is found at the level of the throat and is called the *vishuddha* (see figure 14). It is represented by a circle containing a downward pointing triangle enclosing in its turn a smaller circle. As a lotus it has sixteen petals; its color is brilliant white (or "golden" white); its mantra is the syllable *ham.* The cosmic element governing this center is ether (hence the notion of purity implied in the chakra's name: ether is the most "subtle" of the five elements. Some texts explain the symbolism of the vishuddha by saying that the smaller central circle represents the moon and the triangle within it the yoni, which would mean that we are once again dealing with the male and female principles, here combined in the same intrinsic mode as in the divine hermaphrodite (Shiva, as the Lord who is "half man, half woman").

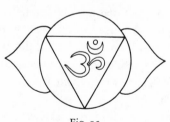

Fig. 15
The ajna

6. The sixth chakra, called the *ajna* (authority), is located at the level of the forehead, between the eyebrows (just above the point where the "third eye" opens) (see figure 15). It is represented by a circle containing a downward-pointing triangle. As a lotus it has two petals only; its color is once more white ("the white of the full moon in all its brilliance"); and its mantra is *om.* The cosmic element related to this center is the one that is placed "above

the five others" and transcends them. Its most usual name is *mahant* (majesty, sovereignty, greatness) and it is likened to the creative power of the Demiurge, though at other times this superelement is said to be the universal intelligence or the world-soul (not brahman but the world's jiva-atman or "incarnate soul"). But in any case, the presence of the syllable *om* within the ajna-chakra's inner triangle is a clear indication that the associated symbolism is that of the origin, the beginning of all things (and that of their end also, since *om* is in equal measure the sonic vibration from which all things emerge and that into which they must eventually be reabsorbed at the end of the cosmic cycle).

7. The seventh and last chakra bears the name *sahasrara,* the thousand-rayed (see figure 16). It is a simple circle of which we are told only that it radiates splendor. As a lotus it naturally has a thousand petals, but it has no specific symbolism (color, sound, or element) connected with it. This is easily understood if we remember that we had already reached the peak of cosmic manifestation with the ajna-chakra: the color white, the syllable *om,* and the element mahant admit of nothing beyond themselves unless it be the Absolute itself, brahman /atman. It must therefore be the Absolute itself that governs the sahasrara, and since "That" (tad) is beyond all quality, it clearly cannot possess any color (unless it be white, which transcends all colors by absorbing them into itself) or any sonority (*om* is a manifestation, a sign of brahman; it cannot strictly speaking be brahman). To attain the sahasrara is thus to attain the "world of brahman (the *brahma-loka,* in which liberation is symbolically "located"). One ought therefore to say that this chakra is located, not "at the top of the head," but rather "above the top of the head," in order to stress that it is differentiated from the other six. The best graphic representations, indeed, show it in the form of an inverted lotus (stem upward, corolla opening downward) emitting a radiance that bathes the subtle body in its entirety (rather like the aura, the golden *vesica piscis* with which Byzantine iconography surrounds the body of Christ).

The symbolism of the chakras is in fact much more complex than my attempt to reduce it to its essentials has made it appear (see table 3). Take the colors, for instance: I have given only the dominant one, the color characteristic of each center as a whole, but it should be realized that each of the chakra's constituent elements (lotus petals, geometric shapes, etc.) has its own particular color. The petals of the muladhara

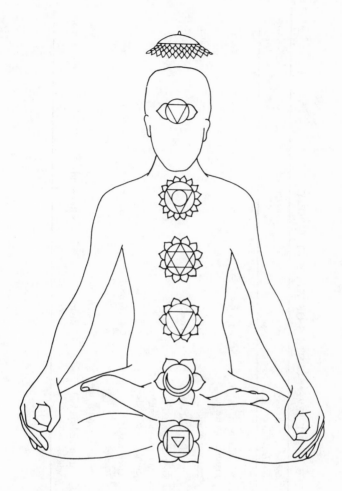

Fig. 16
The sahasrara

are red, for example, like those of the svadhishthana, whereas those of the manipura are golden, and so on. In the same way, the disk of the vishuddha is red, while the triangle and the smaller circle within it are white; the disk of the anahata is red too, but the two triangles are gray, and so on. Nor have I said anything about the letters of the Sanskrit alphabet inscribed on the lotus petals; they symbolize cosmic energy in the form of the revealed word, which by the use of such graphic signs can be transcribed for men's use (though we must remember that in India it is the sound that is of primary importance, not the char-

TABLE 3   THE SEVEN CENTERS OF THE SUBTLE BODY

Name	Location	Geometric shapes inside chakra	Color	Number of lotus petals	Sound	Cosmic power
muladhara	anus	triangle, point down, inside a square	yellow	four	*lam*	earth
svadhishthana	genitals	crescent moon	white	six	*vam*	water
manipura	navel	triangle, point down	red	ten	*ram*	fire
anahata	heart	six-pointed star or "Solomon's seal" made up of two triangles	gray	twelve	*yam*	air
vishuddha	throat	circle inside a triangle	golden white	sixteen	*bam*	ether
ajna	forehead	triangle, point down	moon color	two	*om*	mahant
sahasrara	above head	a thousand-spoked wheel	diamond color	a thousand	—	brahman

acters that represent it). I ought also to have explained that each
center has a presiding deity: Brahma over the muladhara, Vishnu over
the svadhishthana, Rudra (or Agni in his "terrible" shape) over the
manipura, etc. And each god is accompanied by his wife, of course, so
that each chakra has its goddess too. Nor does this exhaust the list
of such details by any means, because Hinduism as we know is passionately fond of subdivisions, refinements, embellishments, analytical
classifications, and tends to feel let down if a symbol is too simple.

However, the essential for us here resides not in the subtleties of
the chakras' symbolism but rather in their function within the subtle
body. The role played by these centers becomes clear at the moment
when the kundalini, rising through the sushumna toward the top of
the head, touches each one on her journey. The texts are fond of saying
that the lotus blossoms in the chakras are normally not more than half-
open buds; they are functioning just enough to sustain the average
individual's ordinary level of existence. For each of the chakras corresponds to a particular form of vital activity: the muladhara presides
over the sense of smell and governs the actions of the lower limbs; the
svadhishthana presides over the sense of taste and governs the actions
of arms and hands; the manipura presides over sight and governs the
excretory organs; the anahata presides over touch and governs the
sexual organs; the vishuddha is in harmony with the sense of hearing
and the mouth; the ajna with all forms of mental activity. Clearly,
then, the kundalini as she ascends is going to cause the lotuses to
blossom and enble their latent energies to manifest themselves with
all the power of which they are capable. This of course is the source
of the miraculous powers described earlier, which, as it has been explained on more than one occasion, are nothing but the perfect realization or fulfillment (siddhi) of natural virtualities, or the unfurling
or blossoming (vibhuti) of those virtualities when finally "realized."

At other times (albeit less often), the texts make use of different
images: they compare the chakras to obstacles that the kundalini
must "break down" or "pierce" in order to reach the seventh center.
The purpose of this approach is to stress the fact that the full realization of a virtuality is at the same time an annihilation of it, since what
is involved, at all six stages, is the transcending of that stage so that
there will be no risk of self-indulgent lingering in it and forgetting
one's ultimate aim, which is liberation. We even find it said on occasion,
as a means of emphasizing the necessity for this transcendence, that

the chakras are actually Gordian knots that the yogi must cut through
with the knife of meditation.

Very little is said about the ascent itself, except that the various
teachers disagree as to whether it is slow, gradual, or rapid (or even
instantaneous). The most traditional schools, following the teaching
of the *Yoga-Sutras,* favor the doctrine that the road is a difficult, arduous one; several attempts are needed, and many yogis will never get
beyond a particular chakra. Other gurus teach the opposite: that once
the kundalini has been awakened and found the entrance to the sushumna, she hurls herself into it and "rearing up like a snake uncoiling
itself in one great leap," reaches the sahasrara right away (or the ajna
at the very least). Knowing how far classical yoga is a school of pa-
tience and endurance, one is inclined to favor the proponents of the
arduous path, yet there is clearly one major objection to their account:
if it is true that samadhi is attained at the moment when the kundalini
reaches the top of the head, then it must follow that those incapable
of drawing it up further than the third or fourth chakra must be forever excluded from that experience. Yet it is difficult to imagine that
a yogi who has succeeded in acquiring total mastery over his body, and
in "dissolving his mind" (by means of dharana), will then prove incapable of practicing meditation with sufficient efficacity to attain
samadhi. The truth (or at least the most widely held opinion) is to be
found between these two extreme positions: most gurus tend to say
that the road leading to sense withdrawal and perfect attention (dharana) is indeed a very difficult one, but that once one has succeeded in
awakening the kundalini, the struggle is essentially over; the power
of the serpent manifests itself in all its strength and samadhi is attained (the adverb "instantaneously" being nugatory here, since the
experience takes place, by definition, outside time).

In Tantric symbolism, samadhi is referred to as the beatific union
of Shiva and his shakti (the goddess Parvati). On the microcosmic level
it is that of the atman (which we must remember is a masculine word
in Sanskrit) and the kundalini, an image of the eternal marriage of
punusha (spirit) and prakriti (nature). And if it is indeed true that
this union knows no end, this means that the yogi who has achieved
this stage "will not return," will never again leave his new status as
a jivan-mukta (liberated-alive):

At the top of the body, above the head,
there is the lotus with a thousand petals,
shining like the light of heaven:
it is the giver of liberation
Its secret name is Kailasa,
the mountain where Shiva dwells.
He who knows this secret place
is freed from samsara.[5]

It is significant that the name Kailasa[6] should be given to this "place outside the body" (sahasrara, the seventh center) in which the yogi finally achieves the goal he first set himself during his noviatiate: liberation (moksha, mukti). For Shiva's paradise is a region of delight where the supreme being (sach-chid-ananda) joys eternally in his union with his shakti: the final liberation is thus presented as being a sort of perpetual wedding feast, an orgasm without end.

This particular coloration of samadhi is specific to Tantrism and is in conformity with the ideology of that movement, which, as we have seen, permeates the whole of modern Hinduism, despite the claims of certain schools that they are completely separate from it. The originality here, as far as yoga is concerned, is that great stress is laid on the contribution of sexual desire to the human composite's motivating force. Of course all schools agree in seeing desire (kama) as the source of the mental impregnations (vasanas) that imprison the soul in the world of phenomena; but most schools seem to "forget," as it were, that the word *kama* has the primary meaning of "love" (eros). Even the *Yoga-Sutras* themselves, in their list of Restraints and Disciplines, mention chastity only once, and then only in passing, as one item among ten others, a sign that in their author's eyes libido was no more than one manifestation, and ultimately a secondary one, of concupiscence in general. Tantrism adopts a diametrically opposed viewpoint: heralding the discoveries of Freud, it places sexual appetite at the center of personality and sees gluttony, craving for wealth, and aggression as derivative forms of that central appetite. From this point of view it is more faithful to the very oldest tradition than the *Yoga-Sutras* are, since it is clearly not just by chance that the term *kama* was selected from among all other possible ones to denote Desire in its universal sense.

If love is indeed the motive force of the world (see above, chapter 5), then its role in the sphere of existence is a preeminent one. Ultimately, one might say that it is indistinguishable from life itself, from nature, from prakriti as cosmic energy. In man, the microcosmic analogue of the universe, love ought similarly to occupy a primary position, both as the determining cause of alienation (which imprisons the individual in the world of phenomena and obliges him to continue transmigrating until the end of the cycle) and as a power capable of liberating him, provided he acquires the necessary intellectual knowledge of his true nature (see above, chapter 6). Thus sexuality, as Nietzsche recognized long since, involves the human being in his entirety, including the domain of spirituality so often thought of as a separate preserve. In which case it is legitimate to make use of sexuality in order to achieve liberation. That is what Tantrism does: taking the old adage that sin itself is a path to salvation, it pushes it to its furthest extremes by teaching that the yogi should eat meat, drink alcohol, and make love to prostitutes, all things forbidden by dharma to high-caste Hindus and viewed by yoga as sins automatically canceling any spiritual progress made. Of course, such practices have no value unless they are directed toward a higher good (salvation, liberation); otherwise they remain sins and certainly serve no purpose (except that of accumulating negative karman). Moreover, the yogi is not permitted to indulge in them until he has undergone his novitiate and reached the stage of sense withdrawal (pratyahara) and perfect concentration (dharana). In other words, these practices are intended to act as aids in the awakening of the kundalini and constitute, in a sense, a form of transcendental meditation (dhyana). And they are also an image of the felicities awaiting the soul (atman) when it has finally achieved liberation from the bonds of existence and is enjoying the ecstasy of union with its shakti.

The omnipresence of the sexual instinct is indicated by seals or geometric figures within the chakras. In this context, however, sexual instinct means a multiform vital energy that can have either male or female manifestations (and it is not the least important aspect of Tantrism that it recognizes the coexistence of both these forms of libido within each and every being, whatever its sex). The feminine element is symbolized, as we have seen, by a downward-pointing triangle, the masculine element by a triangle with point uppermost, or by a representation of the moon (either crescent or circle), or by an erect linga. And we need only turn back to table 3 to see that this double symbolism is clearly apparent in all of the chakras except the seventh, which is of course outside the body. The first two lotuses, for instance, include either the triangle symbolizing the yoni (female sexual organ) or the crescent moon (symbolizing the fertilizing power of the male sexual organ). Moving upward, the lotus at heart level (anahata-chakra) contains both male and female triangles interlocked. And lastly, the ajna-chakra, highest of the "corporeal" lotuses, at forehead level, presents the image of a full moon (male sexual power at its fullest stage of development) enclosing a downward-pointing triangle (the female symbol), and it is here, we are told, that the atman, which resides in this chakra, enters into union with its shakti. The perfection of this union, in the course of which the kundalini is reabsorbed into the atman-purusha (the soul in its male aspect) is the very symbol of love itself ("and they shall be as one flesh," as the Gospel puts it).

The syllable *om* occurring within the last chakra expresses the permanence of this union, its perfection, and its beatific character, while also indicating that its realization will enable the resulting "unitary couple" to attain the thousand-petaled lotus (sahasrara-chakra), where, having once more become one with essence, it will continue forever in blessed solitude (kaivalya or "isolation," the state of the principle of all things, which, because it is one, can have no second). Practitioners of yoga explain that this situation (the eternal marriage of spirit and nature) accounts for the name sach-chid-ananda (being-consciousness-joy) given to the Absolute: the couple *is* for ever, on the level of essence, without any of the limitations of existence; it possesses full consciousness of itself without the slightest distraction; and this full and entire knowledge it has of its eternal marriage is in itself perfect joy or beatitude. When the yogi has attained this ultimate peace (*shanti*) by returning to the principle of all things, then he has reached the goal he set himself at the outset of his quest: the prize is won, and worth all the struggle it has cost.

Conclusion

he limitation of space has obliged me to keep strictly to essentials and to leave certain aspects of yoga unexplored—secondary aspects, it is true, but still of interest. For instance, I have been unable to give any account of the bonds (*bandha*) and seals (*mudra*) that play a part in hatha-yoga even though they are unknown in classical yoga. Rather than wander off into long digressions I preferred to leave these practices to one side, since they are ultimately no more than variants of the classical postures (asanas), and it is perfectly possible to explain yoga, or even practice it, from initiation right through to samadhi, without them. Indeed, a great many texts omit any mention of them. As for Tantrism, to which I have devoted three chapters, it would require a whole volume to do it justice, so rich and complex is the symbolism it employs, and so important are the patterns of thought it has introduced into the whole fabric of modern Hinduism. Nevertheless, I have tried to make clear the place it occupies in the teachings of yoga.

The necessity to be brief does, however, have its advantages: it forces one to choose from among a number of possibilities. I could have elected to stress the picturesque aspect of the subject and provided long lists of postures gleaned from hatha-yoga manuals such as the *Gheranda-Samhita* or the *Hatha-Yoga-Pradipika,* but many other authors have already done that, with lavish aid from drawings and photographs. The theory of the subject, on the other hand, is more often than not passed over in complete silence, even though it is the very foundation of yoga, including the exercises. Would it not be better, I thought, simply to explore the teachings of the basic texts, respecting the relative positions adopted by the doctrine's various branches?

So I decided to allot no more than a modest amount of space to the exercises in order to allow more for an exposition of the underlying doctrine, a choice that has enabled me not only to remain faithful to its founders but also to restore to yoga a dignity that some of the books published in the West during recent decades have succeeded in tarnishing. Yoga, I must repeat, is a darshana, a "way of seeing" Hinduism, just as Vedanta and Tantrism are. It aims first and foremost at explaining the world, at situating man within the universe, at giving him an account of his internal structure, so that it can then go on to offer him a path of spiritual salvation. Once we know what yoga says man is, as well as what he should become, then it is easy to explain that its path to salvation is made up of stages, during which the practitioner must gain mastery over his body. But if one does not know these things, there is a danger of perceiving no more than the exotic value of certain aspects and missing the essential entirely. Ultimately, I believe the reader will not have been disappointed, since the metaphysical system of Patanjali and his successors is a structure on the most magnificent scale, eminently worthy of our admiration.

I explained at the outset of this book that yoga is held by its practitioners to be a doctrine revealed once and for all, at the beginning of the cosmic cycle, by the mythical prophets or rishis, and handed on since that time by word of mouth in accordance with the traditional laws of the master-disciple chain of initiation. So that if there are discrepancies, as there clearly are, between what is taught in the *Bhagavad-Gita,* for example, and present-day practices, this can only be a sign of the gradual erosion of the ancient teachings due to the fact that we live in the last of the cosmic ages, the Iron Age (Kali-Yuga), in which only a quarter of the original knowledge available is still accessible to mankind. We can accept or reject this position, but it is essential that it should first be presented in its most rigorous form, since it is central in the lives of all those yogis today who tell us that the struggles they consent to go through in order to achieve their salvation are justified because they are "prescribed by tradition" and not by such and such an individual. Hinduism—and this is a point worth insisting on—is not only a religion without a founder but also, its followers claim, a religion without a history, since it is after all, in the eyes of its faithful, the *sanatana dharma,* the "eternal norm." Which means that nothing in it has ever changed and that nothing will ever have the power to alter it in any way, even though human weakness may resign itself to living out no more than a small proportion of its commandments. This profoundly Hindu feeling that man is defined by reference to an immutable Absolute must be clearly understood before we can enter into any Western-style investigation of yoga's development.

The first piece of evidence available to anyone wishing to examine yoga historically is the famous representation of an individual sitting cross-legged amidst a number of animals and hieroglyphics. This representation occurs on an earthenware seal that dates from the third millennium B.C. and belongs to the Indus Valley (or Mohenjo-Daro) civilization.[1] The hieroglyphics above the figure's head have not yet been deciphered, so that we still cannot identify him for certain, but it is probable that he is in fact a "proto-Shiva," an identification that seems to be confirmed by the hairstyle, the escort of wild animals, and, above all, the god's posture, which recalls that of a yogi (we know that Shiva is the Great Yogi). Since the Indus Valley civilization preceded the arrival of the Aryans (or Indo-Europeans) into India, it has sometimes been concluded that yoga is non-Aryan; but this is to ignore the fact that Indo-European rituals included techniques for breath control and meditation that were also those of yoga. We know, for example, that the Celts had developed such practices (and a concomitant theory) before Christianity appeared to stamp them out.

In India, where there is no break in the cultural continuity, we can still trace without difficulty the transition from the *Veda* proper (in which there is a famous hymn to "the Long-Haired One") to the *Upanishads* and on to the *Bhagavad-Gita,* in which yoga is presented under its own name, without a mask, as it were. Nevertheless, it must be observed that a decisive divergence becomes apparent at this point (in the sixth century B.C.). Whereas the *Veda,* as well as the normative texts (*Dharma-shastras*) that develop it, expressly advocate life in the world, performance of the duties appropriate to one's condition in it, and achievement of immortality through devout worship and the meticulous performance of required rites, yoga teaches that one must renounce the world and abandon family and home in order to achieve a salvation that is no longer mere immortality within a cycle but a once-and-for-all emergence from the sphere of existence and a reabsorption into the Absolute. The tension between these two currents of thought is apparent in the stringency of the prescriptions aimed at protecting normal society from any contact with sadhus (those who have renounced it). Yet there are also a number of texts (notably the *Bhagavad-Gita*) that strive to bridge the gap by inserting the two rival methods into a hierarchy: devotion and ritual worship are for everyone;

renunciation and yoga are solely for those who feel themselves called. Hence the yogi's paradoxical situation, which still obtains today: although honored, even venerated, he is also the object of a strict ostracism that forbids his being received in orthodox homes.

It is also worth noting, albeit only in passing (since this book is only concerned with the Hindu tradition proper), that the teachings of Buddhism, which arose in India at this time (the sixth century B.C.), are strangely similar to those of yoga: striving toward nirvana (as opposed to paradise), invitation to enter monastic life (i.e., to renounce the world), rejection of the caste system, etc. Indeed, some kind of meeting between yoga and early Buddhism certainly took place, and one of the Buddhist schools is actually called yogachara (practice of yoga). We also know that as Indian Buddhism spread throughout Asia (before disappearing from India itself in about the eighth century after Christ), some ideas from yoga were carried with it into Tibet, Mongolia, China, and from there on into Japan. Indeed, *zen* is a specific form of yoga's dhyana or "transcendental meditation," and the very word "zen" (like its Chinese equivalent *tchan*) is a simple phonetic development from Sanskrit *dhyana.*

To return to India, suffice it to say that the first systematic exposition of yoga is attributed to a certain Patanjali, about whom we know virtually nothing.[2] His work (if it was in fact his) consists of a chain of aphorisms (*sutra*) providing instruction in yoga in a concise, abrupt form that lays all its emphasis upon the doctrinal, metaphysical aspect rather than upon the practical exercises employed to assist the attainment of salvation.

Patanjali's work was later vastly extended by a series of commentaries and a number of independent treatises directly inspired by his teaching. Now that these various texts have been systematically collated, and their language (always Sanskrit but at differing linguistic levels) subjected to philological scrutiny, scholars incline to think that Patanjali lived slightly before Christ, with his principal commentator, Vyasa, following him very closely in time. Later (perhaps between the eighth and ninth centuries), came another great commentary by Vachaspati Mishra, expanded in its turn by a text composed in the ninth century by Bhoja. The interesting point about this line of descent is that it keeps itself aloof from the Tantric current of thought. Tantrism had already begun to produce major works that Mishra and Bhoja decided to ignore, thus inaugurating an attitude that was to perpetuate itself into our own times in works such as those of Vijnana Bhikshu (six-teenth century) and Ramananda Sarasvati (seventeenth century). All these authors share a concern to keep yoga (consequently referred to as "classical" yoga) closely in line with the Patanjalian tradition, which, like the *Bhagavad-Gita,* excludes all mention of the theory of the chakras (centers of the subtle body), the kundalini, and so on.

The earliest written evidence we have of the Tantrist current of thought apparently dates back no further than the tenth century after Christ. Here again, it is clear that such evidence was preceded by a long tradition and did not spring up from nowhere. In India, it must be repeated, no one ever decided to write anything down unless they were prompted by a feeling that the doctrine in question was in danger of being lost or led astray. Therefore, although the first *Tantras* and the first *Yoga Upanishads,* for instance, date from the eighth century after Christ, we may and should assume as a certainty that their contents were formulated at least ten centuries earlier, then continuously elaborated upon and renewed before being finally fixed in the texts we possess. The Vedic pantheon already included female deities, and the earliest form of Brahmanism (several centuries before Christ) allotted an important place to worship of the Goddess in all her forms: Lakshmi (Vishnu's consort), Parvati, Uma, Durga (the names of Shiva's con-sort), Shri (goddess of fortune), Kali (the goddess in her terrible aspect), etc. The notion of shakti (cosmic energy or power) and prakriti (nature) also appears in the texts produced by the various great schools of thought (darshanas), and even the *Bhagavad-Gita* has to take it into account. Nevertheless, it is not until we come to a particular series of *Upanishads* and the first of the *Tantras* that we find the doctrine of the subtle body—with its nadis (channels) and chakras (centers)—clearly formulated, together with that of the kundalini, the feminine force present in all beings regardless of their sex. And it is also from this point onward that we find liberation assimilated into the notion of the eternal marriage between purusha (spirit) and prakriti (nature), represented in its turn as the eternal union of the god (Shiva or Vishnu) and the goddess (Parvati or Lakshmi).

These are the only elements of Tantrism that the many sects make use of in the field of yoga. There is no room here to cite all such sects, but one might mention the Nathas (or Siddhas) whose founder is said to have been a certain Gorakhnath, who probably lived in North-ern India in about the tenth century after Christ. Then there are the

Sahajiyas, in Bengal and Assam, who must be placed on the outer fringes of orthodoxy on account of the relations they maintain with the Moslems on the one one hand and with the Tibetan Buddhists on the other. Yoga in their view (in its most extreme Tantric form) transcends all religious differences, and to them it makes no difference whether one calls oneself a Moslem, or a Hindu, or a Buddhist, provided one is operating on a high enough spiritual plane. In practice, however, the Tantrism of both Nathas and Sahajiyas is clearly situated within a Hindu context and has every appearance of obeying a specific form of dharma. Everything in it, in fact (iconography, vocabulary, forms of worship), is resolutely Hindu; and whatever their distant origins may have been, both these movements have undergone the usual process of Brahmanization during recent centuries: texts written in Sanskrit, growing similarity between their practitioners and the traditional sadhu, etc. But at least the size of these two sects, their vitality, and the deep roots they have put down in those regions of India where orthodox spiritual life is at its most intense (Benares, Gaya, etc.) have been a powerful influence in the diffusion of Tantric yoga throughout the whole subcontinent.

That this is so becomes apparent when one examines the modern masters of yoga. Their teachings are always strongly influenced by Tantrism, even when they claim to have derived them from other currents of classical Hinduism (usually the Vedanta school, which over the past two or three centuries has become the "accepted philosophy" of Indian intellectuals).

The most moving of these figures is certainly Ramakrishna (1834–86), a poor brahmin who spent his entire life in his native Bengal not far from Calcutta. He was a simple priest in charge of a small temple to Kali, married, living the life of a good husband and father, when he was suddenly inflamed with a burning devotion to the goddess which soon led him to renounce the world, even though he continued to fulfill his functions as a priest (the temple was in fact no more than a tiny private shrine frequented by a very small number of worshipers). He justified this situation to himself by seeing it as a form of karma-yoga combined with a bhakti-yoga modeled on that preached by Krishna in the *Bhagavad-Gita*. Later, he was initiated by a wandering sadhu and practiced Tantric yoga to some extent (although the fact that his wife had remained with him throughout had already lent his renunciation a certain Tantric coloration). Gradually disciples began to collect around him and receive instruction from him. The most famous of these was Vivekananda (1863–1902), who after his master's death was to spread Ramakrishna's teaching in the West. The unique feature of the ashram formed around Ramakrishna is that it was transformed under Vivekananda's influence into a monastic order. The monks take vows of renunciation and are then free to practice the type of yoga that best suits them individually. The majority follow the "path of works" (they take part in a number of charitable organizations), others devote themselves to scriptural studies (jnana-yoga), but all combine in their great veneration of the vanished master.

The ashram of Shri Aurobindo (1872–1950) was formed in a similar way.[3] As a young man, he returned to his native Bengal at the end of the last century after completing his studies in England. He quickly found a post and a place in social life. Anti-British militancy being common in this milieu at that time, he joined the movement and later became editor of an anti-Establishment newspaper which he named the *Karma-Yogin,* a choice of title indicating his spiritual preoccupations. He was eventually arrested and served a year's prison sentence, during which time he came to realize that he was on the wrong path. As a result of various spiritual experiences he finally decided that he must devote himself exclusively to the quest for the Absolute and withdrew into seclusion in Pondicherry (1910), where he was to spend the last forty years of his life, alone at first, then increasingly surrounded by disciples and assisted by a Frenchwoman who became his helpmeet (venerated within the ashram under the title of "Mother"). The doctrine preached was a synthesis of yogas: the disciple is invited to experience each of the methods of salvation in turn (karma-yoga, bhakti-yoga, etc.), until he finds his own balance in a kind of raja-yoga in which Tantrism has its place (Aurobindo wrote a long poem celebrating cosmic energy, which he called Savitri, "the incitress"). When he reaches the end of his road, then the practitioner will experience divine life.

Even in Aurobindo's lifetime his ashram had already acquired a very rigid structure and buildings to house it had been either purchased or built. This tendency has continuously become more pronounced in the last few years and has now reached the stage of a projected new town (Auroville).

Needless to say, yoga's influence in modern India is far from being limited to those institutions owing allegiance to the memory of Ramakrishna or Aurobindo. On the contrary, there are gurus without number, and ashrams can be counted in thousands. However, my brief account of these two modern giants will have enabled the reader to perceive some of the particular characteristics of their teaching, characteristics that are shared by almost all contemporary gurus, indeed by all of the best known. In the first place is their fidelity to the traditional method of Indian spiritual education: the unit is still a group of disciples around a master, and direct master-disciple contact is alone recognized as truly efficacious.

When the ashram becomes too large, subgroups are constituted under the guidance of the more advanced disciples, although nothing can replace the direct presence of the guru. At Pondicherry, for example, when Aurobindo decided never again to break silence, the principle of the direct disciple-guru encounter was maintained by means of the ceremony of the *darshana* (vision); on set dates, the disciples were admitted to "view" the master, and their contemplation of him was assumed to produce the same benefits as more usual forms of communication (dialogue, lessons). This was, however, an extreme case and made possible only by the fact that the Mother had already taken over the ashram's practical direction.

The other form taken by fidelity to Indian educational tradition is the predominance given to oral instruction. Ramakrishna never wrote a line, and the practical guidance Aurobindo gave his disciples always took the form of private conversations, before he withdrew into silence. His writings certainly contain the essence of his teaching, but they are all Western-style books written for the purpose of spreading his ideas in the intellectual world, not books of instruction in the proper sense of the term. All those who felt themselves "called" after reading the master's works had to come to his ashram to undergo their novitiate before initiation. In the case of the less well-known ashrams it is still the guru's reputation, as always in the past, that attracts the curious to him; rumor of his excellence will have circulated along the pilgrim routes, where sadhus and faithful meet and converse.

In our day, however, things are tending to change: the presence of the British on Indian soil for nearly two centuries, the use of the printing press, the ability to travel of great distances in a short time—all these assist in the rapid diffusion of ideas, in India as well as elsewhere. Aurobindo's thought was thus able to reach a very wide audience, despite the master's seclusion in a tiny town in the extreme

South. In the same way an ascetic like Ramana Maharshi (1879–1950) was able to attract disciples from all over India, even from abroad, as a result of articles describing the originality of his teaching.[4] Examples of this kind are legion.

What is of most interest to us, however, is that modern conditions have made it possible for non-Indians to acquire a knowledge of Hinduism not just through books but also, if they wish, by direct contact. This poses a problem, because dharma forbids the communication of knowledge to anyone not worthy to receive it, and this "worthiness" is defined not merely in moral but primarily in ritual or dogmatic terms: only the "twice-born" or dvijas have rightful access to the scriptures. The dvijas, it will be recalled, are those Hindus who have been admitted to the sacrament of upanayana (a boy's initiation ceremony), which means that no one can receive spiritual instruction unless he is born in India itself to a high-caste family. The enormous mass of shudras (the service castes) and pariahs (outcastes) is excluded from liturgical life, and foreigners even more so!

In other words a Westerner is forbidden to be converted to Hinduism, and contact with the religion would be quite impossible for a Westerner were it not for the existence of certain sects and the ashrams, since the former reject the caste system and are therefore able (theoretically anyway) to accept new members from any background, and the latter are, by definition, open to all. An ashram, as we saw earlier, is in fact a free congregation of sadhus (those who have renounced the world) around a guru who is himself necessarily a sadhu also. Since "renunciation" in Hinduism means first and foremost the rejection of everything that constitutes worldly life, beginning with its social organization (the caste system), there can therefore be no obstacle to the admission of foreigners into any ashram. As we know, many Westerners have traveled to India to be taught by Vivekananda, Gandhi, Ramana Maharshi, Aurobindo, and a great many others. It must be emphasized, however, that this acceptance remains valid only within the restricted boundary of the ashram itself. The moment a foreigner emerges into the world again, he becomes once more the "barbarian" he has never ceased to be in Hindu eyes, and reverts to being a pariah even among pariahs. As may easily be imagined, this can lead to conflicts and disappointments.

However, the fact that so many Westerners still make the journey is not without significance. It is a sign that Hinduism, particularly in the form of yoga, is answering a need. And it would be wrong to think that we are dealing here with a wholly new development, one determined by the conditions of existence in the present-day world. Quite the contrary is true; the "call of the East" dates back for centuries. From the Greeks to Marco Polo, from Vasco da Gama to Dupleix and Warren Hastings, the West has never ceased to dream of the treasures of Golconda, of the land of spices—and of the wisdom of the brahmins. When direct contact was rendered possible by the opening of the sea route around Africa, this fascination was given tangible treasures to feed upon. One has only to think, for instance, of the eighteenth-century craze for printed calicoes (the French called them *indiennes*) and of the fact that the fundamental Hindu scriptural texts actually became accessible in translation during the last years of the same century. Their impact was prodigious: the *Bhagavad-Gita,* the *Upanishads,* and later the *Bhagavata-Purana* produced a tremendous intellectual ferment, particularly in Germany and France. Schopenhauer was fond of saying that the first intuition of the work he was to do came to him while reading these texts, of which he was later to say that they had been "his life's consolation." Aside from Schopenhauer, none of the early nineteenth-century German philosophers (Herder, Schelling, and Hegel especially) failed to find a place for India in their works. And then there were the Romantics! All of them, without exception, were passionately interested in finding out all they could about Indian literature and thought. If one wishes to form an idea of the fervor that things Indian created in Europe at that time, then one has only to read what Goethe, Hugo, Nerval, Lamartine, Blake, Shelley, and many others had to say on the subject. There was not an important work that did not refer in some way to the Indian tradition.

Meanwhile, occultist circles (taking "occultist" in its widest sense) were passionately studying Brahmanic symbolism and the general ideology of classical India, in which they were able to recognize, magnified and clarified, all the basic principles of Western esoteric thought (beginning with the principle of analogy, which constitutes the foundation for all systems of such a kind in whatever sphere—magic, alchemy, yoga, etc.). The impetus of this movement led to the founding of the Theosophical Society, whose influence was to be such a decisive factor in the nineteenth century. It can truly be said that from this point on it was no longer possible to write any work on esoteric thought without taking India into account. The work of men like

René Guenon, Aldous Huxley, A. K. Coomaraswamy, and others is particularly significant in this respect.

Outside these circles, and usually in conflict with them, "official" science had developed an autonomous department within its own establishment devoted to the analysis of Indian culture in all its diversity. For almost two centuries now, philologists, historians, philosophers, sociologists, and ethnologists have been engaged in a vast labor of exploration that has resulted in the publication of tens of thousands of tomes in all the tongues of Europe. For many years, however, this vast mass of research remained largely inaccessible to the general public on account of its extreme technicality, even though translations and a number of general works synthesizing its results did succeed in reaching a certain number of people and maintaining the interest of various highly educated groups. A meager result, when one thinks of the curiosity that exists today about everything that lies beyond the Mediterranean.

Eventually, therefore, the task was taken over by the Hindu teachers themselves. And Vivekananda's travels through America and Europe (as a result of his invitation to the World Parliament of Religions held in Chicago in 1893) remain the standard example of this kind of "mission": lectures, more intimate gatherings in the homes of well-disposed hosts, the composition of a few generalized works, followed very quickly by a number of genuine conversions (the first was that of an aristocratic Englishwoman, Margaret Noble, who became a nun in Ramakrishna's order), so that the guru finds himself obliged to accept foreign disciples. He has usually preferred to do this in his own ashram, in India (as in the case of Ramana Maharshi, Aurobindo, etc.), but nowadays there is an increasing demand on him to come to the West and take a hand in the good work there himself. (Disciples can be very insistent in this respect; arguing that they cannot all totally renounce the world, they are adamant that the guru must come and visit them instead from time to time. This is what Vivekananda did, then his successors (the *swamis* of the Mission Ramakrishna), followed by a great number of other gurus. This is a truly new phenomenon, since the only other known instances we have of Indian culture being exported date back to the earliest centuries of the Christian era, at the time when Buddhism and (secondarily) Hinduism were being spread through central and Southeastern Asia.

Travels on this scale must clearly be the result of a genuinely pressing appeal, emanating from ever broader sections of modern Western society. Let us take an example: the meetings that Vivekananda attended never involved more than a dozen or so people at a time, many of whom were merely sensation-seekers; but in 1971 I myself saw a thousand Westerners (mostly Americans) arriving to take part in a ten-week retreat that was to be held on one of the Balearic Islands in an isolated hotel transformed for that purpose into an ashram around the Maharishi Mahesh Yogi. It was not a "sunshine holiday" they were in for either, but ten weeks of full time, intensive work, in strict seclusion, on a special diet, and so on. The great majority of those present were less than thirty years old and came from middle- or lower-middle-class backgrounds. All or almost all of them were students playing truant from their other courses of study. Three things are new here: the presence of the guru who has left India to visit the West (his ashram is at Rishikesh at the foot of the Himalayas), the large number of disciples, and lastly their age. We are a long way from the traditional picture of the theosophist, the occultist, or any of the other India enthusiasts whom one has tended to think of as elderly folk given to holding small, sedate meetings now and then in a somewhat clubbish atmosphere.

The change began to take place immediately after the war, then accelerated rapidly in the late fifties. This acceleration coincided with the sudden development in America, then in Europe via Britain, of the hippy movement, itself the outcome of various earlier trends, in particular that exemplified by the beatniks. What we are faced with here is the spread of a whole ideology, which, though it may lack a clear and explicit structure, is nonetheless very coherent: a Nietzschean reversal of values (together with the setting up of a counterculture); rejection of society in its present form; the search for any means of exploding set forms of thought, including blowing the mind with hallucinogens; a dionysiac cult of the body; and the desire for perpetual nomadic wandering. Whether rightly or wrongly, Hinduism is invoked as one of its terms of reference (as early as the beatnik days the poet Allen Ginsberg used to invite his audiences to recite mantras with him), though of course it is the marginal forms of Hinduism that are canvassed. The model offered is not the orthodox brahmin, the law-abiding head of a household, but the sadhu who, like the hippy, has rejected worldly values, renounced the social structure of his country, and is leading the life of a wandering beggar in which the use of drugs occasionally plays a part. In both cases the long hair, the conspicuously different clothing, and the spiritual thirst serve as identifying badges. It is certain that the hippies did not adopt their hairstyle in conscious imitation of the sadhus, but like causes everywhere produce like effects; every regimented society wishes its members to cut their hair in accordance with the prevalent canons of fashion, and not to do so is an act of provocation creating a gap that people find hard to bridge between "civilized men" and "savages."

What is new here is this convergence of attitude over such distances in time (because renunciation is hardly a novelty in India) and space. The future alone can tell whether the hippy movement has in fact enabled the West to know India better or whether, on the contrary, the Indian influence on certain sectors of Western youth is no more than a fleeting and superficial phenomenon.

As for yoga itself, it could hardly fail to benefit from this vogue, since all sadhus are practitioners of it. Here again there is a marked contrast between present-day and earlier attitudes. Theosophy, occultist circles, and "official" Indianists were all aware of yoga's existence, but they allowed it no more than a secondary importance. It is remarkable, for instance, that no important work was written about it before the present century. Vivekananda's preaching always remained very theoretical, and Romain Rolland, though he devoted three whole volumes to Ramakrishna and Vivekananda, left the practical aspect of the discipline wholly unexplored. It would be interesting to know exactly when the first "schools of yoga," teaching the postures and breath control, were founded in the West. Unless I am much mistaken, it cannot have been before the First World War, and it was not until the late fifties that such establishments appeared in any number or —even more to the point— achieved any success among large sectors of the population.

It is unnecessary to repeat here what I said at the outset of this book about the yoga "craze" we are going through in the West, though I would like the reader to understand that I intend no value judgment in what I have already said. My aim has been simply to state facts that are accessible to anyone who really wishes to know them and think about them. Yoga is a complete and perfectly structured world view that requires both an unqualified adherence and a long apprenticeship; that is something clearly stated by the texts and continualy repeated by the yoga masters. To refuse such adherence, to sort through the practices and theories of yoga, picking and choosing what we feel suits us, is an attitude we undoubtedly have the right to adopt, but it is one that places us outside yoga itself. Perhaps it would be better to impregnate ourselves first, sympathetically and attentively, with the ideology of yoga, with its theory, before deciding whether or not we wish to devote ourselves to its practice. The sole aim of this book has been to make such a course possible, as far as lay within my power.

Yoga Darshana Upanishad

INTRODUCTION

among the Hindu scriptures dealing with yoga, the *Upanishads* stand somewhat apart and play what is in many respects a paradoxical role. For one thing, the Brahmanic tradition treats them as an integral part of the *Veda,* yet it is quite clear, even to an orthodox pandit, that they have very close links with non-Vedic texts such as the *Bhagavad-Gita* or the *Yoga-Sutras.* One has the impression that they were written (by anonymous authors at unknown dates) solely in order to provide a "Vedic seal of approval" for what were really "modern" (that is, post-Vedic) teachings. Very probably they were the product of what amounted to "yoga academies" formed around gurus of high reputation and made up of followers from the most diverse backgrounds (since we know that caste differences were usually ignored in such ashrams). In such a situation it would not be surprising if the literate brahmins among a master's following should have conceived the idea of preserving his teaching in short compositions of this kind. Since they would have revered their gurus no less than they did the greatest rishis (prophets) of the Vedic scriptures, why should they not have given these collections of "lecture notes," as it were, the form, sacred among all others, of the *Upanishad?*

The more so since the *Upanishad* as a literary genre was a particularly suitable one for their purpose. The typical *Upanishad* excludes philosophical argument; the dialogues in them are fictitious (except possibly in the case of the two oldest: the *Chandogya* and the *Brihad-Aranyaka,* which are exceptional on more than one count); the truth (that is, the writer's opinion) is presented in a peremptory manner with the aid of numerous curt phrases such as "there is no doubt that . . ."; and if any opinion at variance with the guru's happens to be mentioned, then it is only in order to attribute it to "the ignorant," whose errors are ridiculed and pitied.

All these characteristics are precisely those to be found in the traditional ashrams, particularly in those easily observable today. It is a rule that the guru shall be regarded as a god: disciples prostrate themselves before him and content themselves with whatever lessons he is kind enough to grant them; no one would dream for an instant of raising a doubt, and even less of actually arguing with him. Anyone who is dissatisfied with the instruction he is receiving simply leaves the ashram without further ado, since there can be absolutely no question of "dialogue" or "seminars" in these institutions, only of the imparting of truth in the form chosen by the master, for reasons that concern no one but himself. When the guru speaks, he does so in the same way as a priest delivering a sermon, or a moral preceptor giving instructions. And he is heard in total humility. Moreover, this becomes even more true where yoga teaching proper is concerned; blind obedience to the guru is one of the "qualities" required of the novice, and Indian literature has a particular fondness for stories about disciples falling into the hands of sadistic or absent-minded masters who make use of a poor aspirant simply as a personal servant, sometimes for years on end, while "forgetting" his very existence!

The *Upanishads* thus provide a faithful reconstruction of the devout atmosphere that existed in such ashrams, where the disciples vied with one another in submissiveness and humble fervor. It should be added that they display no evidence of a concern for literary quality. They are composed for the most part in *shlokas,* very loosely constructed stanzas of four octosyllabic lines each, which are used for the sole purpose of helping novices to memorize them by rote more easily (the actual spiritual content being injected later by the oral commentaries of the master or his principal disciples). The composition as a whole tends to be rather slipshod; groups of shlokas are often found out of their natural context, while others are sometimes repeated word for word. The general plan is rarely well balanced, and it is not unusual to find sections that are four or five times longer— for no good reason—than others that are at least as interesting or important.

Even as they stand, however, these short compositions are still of great documentary interest. In the field of yoga, for instance, they reveal aspects of the doctrine that we would hardly have suspected if the *Upanishads* had not existed. Neither the *Bhagavad-Gita* nor the *Yoga-Sutras* makes any mention of the chakras, for example, or of the kundalini, and it is fortunate for us that the *Yoga Upanishads* allot them the space that they deserve in the general structure of yoga theory (for without them, how would we understand exactly what happens during deep meditation—dhyana—to trigger its mutation into samadhi?).

As an example of texts of this kind I have chosen the *Yoga-Darshana,* one of the most characteristic. The text on which I have based my translation is that published by Adyar (Madras, 1952). The *Yoga Darshana Upanishad* (or simply *Darshana Upanishad,* as it is possible to call it in the context of a collection devoted solely to the *Yoga Upanishads*) is a text of classical composition in the sense that the material to be taught is dealt with in its natural order, the same one as that employed in the *Yoga-Sutras*: the eight rungs of yoga are diligently climbed in ascending sequence, one by one. Nevertheless, at various points we find that the authors have inserted lessons on matters not dealt with by the *Yoga-Sutras*. For instance, we find that the *Upanishad* interposes an account of the nadis (channels for the circulation of the "vital" or subtle breath) between its description of the various yoga positions and that of breath control techniques (pranayama); and a very logical position this is, for it is the theory of how the vital breath circulates through the nadis that makes pranayama comprehensible. Similarly, a long section on the geography of the subtle body (with its mountains, its rivers, its places of pilgrimage) is inserted to clarify the benefits derived from the practice of pranayama. Such digressions are typical of the *Upanishads*—compositions more concerned with theory than with practice, and intended by their very nature to be presentations of the ideological foundation of yoga technique (in the case of the *Yoga Upanishads*) rather than meticulous descriptions.

This becomes clear from an analysis of the content of the *Yoga Darshana Upanishad.* The work is made up of ten *khandas* (main sections or chapters) of extremely unequal length:

the first (25 shlokas) describes the restraints (yamas);
the second (16 shlokas) gives a list of the disciplines (niyamas);
the third (13 shlokas) describes a number of the simpler positions (asanas);
the fourth (63 shlokas) describes the geography of the subtle body and the system of nadis;

the fifth (14 shlokas) is an extension of the fourth and explains the
procedure for inner purification;

the sixth (51 shlokas) sets out a detailed theory of breath control
(pranayama);

the seventh (14 shlokas) deals with sense withdrawal (pratyahara);

the eighth (9 shlokas) is concerned with dharana, the fixing of attention on a single point;

the ninth (6 shlokas) deals briefly with deep meditation (dhyana);

the tenth and last (12 shlokas) is a conclusion preceded by a eulogy
of samadhi, the ultimate stage of yoga in which the soul achieves
identity with the Absolute.

One is struck by the disproportionate lengths of these various chapters: a bare six stanzas on dhyana and more than sixty devoted to describing the nadis. Ten stanzas on samadhi as opposed to fifty on
breath control. Clearly this cannot just be the result of chance. Probably the authors of the *Upanishad* decided it would be pointless to repeat
the clear and precise instructions on technical points provided by the
Yoga-Sutras but believed that they ought to pass on their own guru's
supplementary commentaries on them. Let us take an example: the
eighth chapter, the one devoted to dharana (fixing attention on a
single point), says nothing about the technique to be employed in
achieving this mental immobility (despite its great difficulty), but
instead instructs the aspirant that he will be well advised to employ
dharana (with which he is assumed to be familiar) in order to recognize in his body the presence of the five elements and their guardian
gods. Here, as in every other case, the *Upanishad* is choosing to offer
instruction that is parallel or complementary to that contained in the
basic texts available to everyone. And in doing so it is undoubtedly
recording for us the original lessons of the master who presided over
its composition.

The interest of the *Yoga Darshana Upanishad* therefore resides
essentially in these esoteric theories (communicated solely to properly
initiated disciples) concerning the anatomy of the subtle body (the
nadis) and its analogy with the geography of the earth: the channels
through which the breath circulates are rivers, all possessing their
appropriate sacred fords (*tirthas*). These places of pilgrimage, frequented on earth by the devout of the various Hindu obediences, take
the form within the subtle body of privileged points that must be rec-

ognized with the help of one's guru. By guiding one's breath to them, one obtains inner purification, which is obviously even more important than outward purification. However, the technique is analogous in both, since the breath is conceived of as making a pilgrimage from tirtha to tirtha just as worshipers do on earth. And just as those worshipers bathe themselves in the water of the sacred fords, so the breath is bathed in the water of the inward tirthas. Only the inward water is no longer that of the Ganges but, as the *Upanishad* says, "the water of the knowledge imparted by the master."

Equally interesting is the fact that the *Yoga Darshana Upanishad* is at pains to reconcile yoga with *Vedanta:* the text's leitmotiv is that the atman is identical with brahman, and that the latter, since it is pure essence, absolutely transcends the phenomenal world. Ultimately, indeed, one can say that the very existence of the universe is brought into question, since the authors claim that there is no phenomenal world at all (10.3)—an extreme position that leads them directly to a negation of all that is not brahman and the statement that transmigration itself is nothing but an illusion without true reality. This being so, the "fruit" of yoga lies in the awareness its practitioner achieves —by meditation and all the other practices leading to samadhi—that nothing exists (outside brahman, which "is" as immutable essence). If he succeeds in this, he enters the state of absolute solitude (kaivalya) that the earlier *Yoga-Sutras* likewise stated to be the ultimate goal of those who enter on the path of yoga. In other words, after following the path of *Vedanta* for part of the way, the *Upanishad* finally returns to the orthodox doctrine of the great yoga texts, just as the *Bhagavad-Gita* does in the end, even though it, too, first takes the opposite path of advocating devotion to a personal god as a precondition of yoga practice. The study of such texts thus enables us to appreciate at once the diversity of the possible approaches and their underlying unity. And to do that is to recognize one of the constants in classical Hindu thought and belief.

Yoga Darshana Upanishad

1.1   The great yogi Dattatreya,
the magnanimous Lord, it is he,
Vishnu,[1] the Great, with four arms,
who reigns as sovereign
over the science of yoga.

1.2   Now his favorite disciple,
Samkriti Maharshi, one day
when he was alone with his holy guru,[2]
bowing before him,
questioned him, his hands pressed together
as a sign of respect!

1.3   "Teach me, Lord,
this science of yoga,
complete with its eight stages,
since I know that by understanding it
I shall become a liberated-alive!"

1.4   Vishnu answered him:
"Listen well, Samkriti,
I will explain yoga to you!

1.5   "Restraints, spiritual disciplines,
postures, breath control,
withdrawal of the senses, and perfect attention,
meditation, and final enstasis,
these are the eight steps!

1.6   "To resolve not to harm any being,
not to lie, not to steal,
to remain chaste and have pity,
to live in equanimity and without weakness,

firm in your beliefs,
without gluttony and always clean,
such are the ten restraints.

1.7   "Not to do any ill to any being
in act, in word, in thought,
that is ahimsa according to the *Veda,*
for the atman is present everywhere,
inaccessible to the senses, in all beings:
recognizing atman in them, that is true ahimsa
those who know have said.

1.9   "The real is what one perceives
by one's sight, by hearing, by the other senses,[3]
since all that exists is brahman,
as those who know say.

1.11   "Ceasing to covet in thought
the wealth of others, whether it be straw,
gold, jewel, or pearl, that is righteousness;
and in atman not to see its contrary,
that is more righteous still:
so say those who know.

1.13   "By abstaining from contact with women,
in act, in word, in thought,
and even from contact with your own wife
except in the days following her periods,
you will be practicing chastity,
applying your mind, without distraction,
to the quest for brahman.

1.14   "To have pity is to see your fellow man,
in act, in word, in thought,
just as though he were yourself:
thus say those who know.

1.15   "To behave in exactly the same way
toward any person whatever,

son, friend, wife, enemy,
always: that is equanimity.

1.16   "Not to yield to the weakness
of becoming enraged against your enemies,
even should they provoke you:
that is the eighth restraint.

1.17   "Knowledge is wakened into life
by renunciation of the world
and study of the scriptures;
to know that is to be firm,
and to have faith
in what the *Veda* states:
'I am atman, and nothing more!'

1.19   "To keep gluttony at bay,
leave on the tray a quarter
of the food served to you:
in this way you will make progress
in your journey toward yoga.

1.20   "And keep your body clean
by rubbing it with clay and water:
in this way you will purify the outside;
but do not forget purity of mind
which consists in knowing that one is pure
in the depths of oneself, since the atman is pure
while the body is impure;
anyone who forgot that, even though keeping his body
      washed,
would lose everything, like the madman
ignoring the gold and taking a clod of earth instead!

1.23   "The yogi who sates himself
with the ambrosia of knowledge
after saying farewell to the world
has no duties left to fulfill;

if he thought he had,
then he would have no right to the name of 'sage.'

1.25   "Yes, to know the atman
is to know that there is nothing
that is worth doing in the world:
and so, through the Restraints, one must
learn to know the atman
as identical with the immutable brahman.

2.1   "Now here are the spiritual disciplines:
ascesis and contentment,
belief in the real, knowing how to give,
devotion, faith in the scripture,
humility and self-abandonment,
constant prayer and observance;
these I will now explain to you.

2.2   "Ascesis, the sages have said,
is to fast at the prescribed times
in order to mortify oneself.
But deeper still is the ascesis of the mind
when one searches for the 'why?'
and for the 'how?' of transmigration
and the means of liberating oneself from it.

2.3   "It is certainly good
to be content with what one earns,
day by day, as the chance of life dictates;
but much better is the contentment
one enjoys through renunciation,
until one knows brahman.

2.6   "By the scriptures and by the tradition
one can be sure that the world exists:[4]
that is what the sage calls
belief in the real.

2.7   "As for knowing how to give,
         that means distributing
         to wise men versed in the scriptures
         what one has justly earned
         or whatever one receives by chance,
         without having sought it.

2.8   "When the heart has freed itself
         from covetousness and the passions,
         when one speaks without lying,
         when one acts without violence,
         then one can say one is practicing
         devotion in truth.

2.9   "As for faith in the scripture,
         that means believing in the reality of the world,
         in infinite knowing,
         in perpetual joy,
         and in the permanence of brahman.

2.10   "Humility is to be ashamed
         of any action that the *Veda*
         or the laws of custom
         declare to be bad, and that one has performed
         from weakness of character.

2.11   "To abandon self is to believe
         without any reservation or doubt
         in what the scriptures teach,
         and to hold to that belief whatever happens,
         even if your guru tries
         to make you believe something different![5]

2.12   "Constant prayer
         is prescribed by the *Veda*,
         the *Books of Ritual*, the *Puranas*,
         the *Dharma-Shastras*, and the *Epics*.

2.13   "One can pray in two ways:
         aloud, or in silence;

And if one prays with words,
it can be out loud or quietly;
and if one prays mentally,
it can be in a murmur,
or else by meditation.

2.15   "And indeed, by praying in a clear voice
one earns the benefits
promised by the scriptures,
but murmured prayer
is more powerful still.

2.16   "As for mental prayer,
it is said to be a thousand times more efficacious,
for you know well that the mantras
no longer give their expected fruits
if by misfortune pariahs should hear them;
and so one must pray mentally.[6]

3.1   "Listen now
to the way of holding the nine positions:
the auspicious sign, the muzzle,
the lotus, the hero, and the lion,
the prosperous and the liberated,
the peacock and the good fortune.

3.2   "Hold yourself very straight, head high,
cross your legs in the proper manner
tucking your feet into the hollows
behind your bent knees: this is the position
called the auspicious sign.

3.3   "If you sit directly
on top of both ankles, that is the muzzle.

3.4   "And if you place both feet
soles upward, on your thighs,
right hand holding the toes of the left foot,
left hand holding the toes of the right foot,

that is the lotus position
By means of which one overcomes sickness.

3.6   "Hold yourself upright in a standing position,
then bend back your left leg
so that the left foot touches your right thigh:
that is the position of the hero.

3.7   "If you bend your legs at the knees
without crossing them and place your heels
against the perineum with your hands
holding your feet in place,
that is the prosperous position.

3.8   "But if you modify
the position of your feet
so as to cross them against the perineum,
that becomes the liberated position.

3.9   "Placing your hands flat on the ground,
elbows bent at the level of the navel,
raise your body horizontally
head held very straight and body stretched out
like a wand: that is the peacock.

"As for those weak of body, let them take up
any relaxed position:[7]
that position will be the good fortune position for them.

3.12   "One must work hard at the positions,
because if one makes oneself absolute master of them,
one will reign over the three worlds;
but then one must try to master
the practice of breath control.

4.1   "The measure of the body
is ninety-six finger's breadths:
in its center there burns a great fire,
bright as molten gold.

4.2   "Two finger's breadths from the anus,
        just below the genitals, is a triangle;[8]
        so teach those who know.

4.3   "As for the knot-of-the-navel,[9]
        that is found in the center of the body,
        nine finger's breadths from the muladhara;
        its diameter is four finger's breadths;
        it resembles a chicken's egg;
        it is enveloped in a sheath, and the navel proper
        is visible in the center of it.

4.6   "In the knot-of-the-navel
        the sushumna is situated
        and seventy-two thousand[10] nadis
        radiate from her, oh Samkriti!
        Fourteen alone are important:

4.7   "the sushumna, the pingala,
        the ida and the sarasvati,
        and the nadis pusha, varuna, hastijihva,
        yashasvini, alambasa,
        kuhu, vishvadara, payasvini,
        shankhini and gamdhara.

4.9   "But three count above all:
        the sushumna, ida, and pingala,
        the most important of all
        being by far the sushumna,
        which adepts of yoga
        call the brahma-nadi.[11]

4.11   "Two finger's breadths below the navel
        resides the kundalini
        formed of earth and the waters,
        of fire, of air, and of ether,
        of thought and intelligence
        as well as of personality.[12]

4.13   "It is she who controls
            the action of the ten vital breaths[13]
            and the assimilation of food,
            in the region of the knot-of-the-navel;
            coiled round upon herself, she keeps her mouth
            upon the hole-of-brahman.[14]

4.14   "To her left is ida;
            pingala rises on her right.

4.15   "On either side of the sushumna
            are kuhu and sarasvati.
            The gamdhara and the hastijihva
            flank the ida before and behind,
            themselves doubled by varuna,
            pusha and the yashasvini;
            the shankhini doubles the gamdhara.
            Lastly, stretched from anus to navel,
            one finds the alambasa.

4.18   "Parallel to the sushumna,
            the color of the full moon, is the kuhu.
            ida and pingala rise as far as the nose,
            to the level of the two nostrils.
            The yashasvini reaches down to the toes of the left foot;
            the pusha runs up to the left eye,
            parallel with the pingala.

4.20   "Payasyini reaches up to the right ear
            and the sarasvati to the tongue;
            the hastijihva runs down to the toes of the right foot
            and the shankhini to the right ear.
            Lastly, the gamdhara reaches up to the right eye,
            while the vishvadara
            remains in the knot-of-the-navel.

4.23   "There are ten vital breaths,
            to which yogis give these names:
            prana, apana, vyana,

samana, udana, naga,
kurma and krikara,
devadatta, dhanamjaya.

4.24   "Of these ten, five are important:
prana, apana, vyana,
udana, samana; but again,
of these five two are foremost:
prana and apana, to which
worship is accorded by the great yogis;
but prana remains the first of them all.

4.26   "Prana is omnipresent:
in the throat, in the nose, in the navel,
in the heart, there it resides permanently;

4.27   "apana, for its part, inhabits
the anus, the thighs and the knees,
the lower part of the body up to the navel;

4.28   "vyana is in the head,
the ears, the eyes, the neck,
down to the level of the shoulders;

4.29   "udana inhabits the limbs
and samana the whole body;
the five other vital breaths
reside in the skin, the bones, and the flesh.

4.30   "The role of prana
is to regulate breathing and coughing;
that of apana the excretions;
vyana produces sounds;
samana gathers together, and udana
enables the body to rise: that is the teaching.

4.33   "Naga causes belching;
dhanamjaya fills the belly;
kurma causes the eyes to close,

and hunger comes through krikara;
as for devadatta, oh Samkriti,
it is the vital breath that brings us sleep.

4.35   "The gods reign over the nadis:
the god of the sushumna is Shiva,
Vishnu is the god of the ida,
and Brahma of the pingala;

"to Viraj is subject the sarasvati,
to Pushan the nadi pusha,
and to Vayu the varuna;

"the hastijihva to Varuna,
the yashasvini to the sun;
Varuna also protects the alambusa
and the god of hunger kuhu;
the moon reigns over the two nadis
gamdhara and shankhini,
Prajapati over the payasvini,
and Soma over the vishvadara.

4.39   "In ida the moon moves,
and in pingala the sun;
that is why when the prana
of pingala enters ida,
that is said to be the northern path;[15]
while the southern path, on the other hand,
is when the breath goes from ida into pingala.

"The moon and the sun unite
within your body when the breath
resides in the meeting place
of the two nadis ida and pingala.[16]

4.43   "It is the spring equinox
when the breath is in the muladhara.
and it is the autumn equinox
when the breath is in the head.

"And prana, like the sun,
travels through the signs of the zodiac;
each time you inhale,
hold in your breath before expelling it.

4.46   "Lastly, an eclipse of the moon
occurs when the breath reaches
the abode of kundalini
via the channel ida,
and when it follows pingala
in order to reach kundalini,
then there is an eclipse of the sun!

4.48   "The Mount Meru is in the head
and Kedara[17] in your brow;
between your eyebrows, near your nose,
know, dear disciple, that Benares stands;
in your heart is the confluence
of the Ganges and the Yamuna;[18]
lastly, Kamalalaya[19]
is to be found in the muladhara.

"To prefer 'real' tirthas[20]
to those concealed in your body,
is to prefer common potsherds
to diamonds laid in your hands.

4.51   "Your sins will be washed away,
whether you have made love with your wife
or even with your own daughter,
if you carry out the pilgrimages
within your own body from one tirtha to another!

"True yogis
who worship the atman in themselves[21]
have no need of water tirthas
or of gods of wood and clay.

"The tirthas of your body

infinitely surpass those of the world,
and the tirtha-of-the-soul is the greatest of them:
the others are nothing beside it.

4.54   "The mind, when sullied,
cannot be purified
in the tirthas where man bathes himself,
any more than a pot containing alcohol
can ever be purified with water,
even though you were to wash it a hundred times!

"Yet the water of knowledge
imparted by the masters of yoga
will purify the sullied mind,
for it is that of a true tirtha!

4.57   "Shiva resides in your body;
you would be made to worship him
in images of stone or wood,
with ceremonies, with devotions,
with vows or pilgrimages.

4.58   "The true yogi looks into himself,
for he knows that images
are carved to help the ignorant
come nearer to the great mystery![22]

"The only true seer
is he who sees brahman,
the real, the one without second,
as identical with his own atman.

4.60   "And then, through renunciation,
you will realize: 'I am the atman';
then you will see that the atman
resides in the depth of all beings;
and the vision of the all-powerful,
the supreme, imperishable brahman,
will deliver you from all pain.

5.1 "Having achieved a correct attitude
to the teaching of the scriptures,
having purged away all concupiscence
and learned what yoga is,
with a serene and truthful mind
you will now be able to enter upon the Path.

5.3 "Lean for strength upon your atman,
listen well to what the masters teach;
go to live in an ashram
situated in a pleasant spot
at the very top of a hill
or on the banks of a river
or else in the forest
not far from a stand of *bilva*,[23]
and practice the postures,
taking care to keep your body straight,
without moving, mouth closed.
Fixing your eyes on the end of your nose,
you will see the disk of the moon there,
distilling ambrosia, drop by drop.

5.7 "Guiding the inhaled air,
through the ida, down into your belly,
meditating on the fire burning
in the center of your body, you will perceive
within yourself the eternal Sound;[24]
then you will expel the air
through the channel of the pingala.

5.10 "Then you will do the same thing again,
but replacing ida with pingala:
continue to practice this at least three times a day,
six breaths in and out each time.

5.11 "In this way you will succeed
in purifying your nadis:
your body will become luminous,

resplendent with the inner fire,
and you will hear the Sound clearly.

5.12   "Then you must
purify the atman itself.
Because in fact, though eternally pure,
luminous and made of joy,
your atman is, as it were, tarnished,
sullied, by the dirt of ignorance.

5.14   "Thanks to true knowledge,
you will be able to remove the mud
and restore its purity.

6.1   "Now comes control of the breath:
you must know that the three stages
that lend rhythm to your breathing
are no other than the separate sounds
that make up the pranava.[25]

"When you guide the air down
into your belly through the ida,
meditate on the letter *A*
for a count of at least sixteen.

"When you hold the air inside you,
meditate on the letter *U*
for a count of at least sixteen,
while allowing *om* to sound within you.

"And when you expel the air
through the channel of the pingala,
meditate on the letter *M,*
trying to protract the process for a count of thirty-two:
that is the true pranayama.

6.7   "Guide the air down once more
through the channel of the pingala,
meditating on the letter *A*
for a count of at least sixteen.

"Then hold the air inside you,
meditating on the letter *U*
and doing your best to hold the air in
for a count of sixty-four
while repeating the pranava.

"And finally, expel the air
using the channel of the ida
meditating on the letter *M*
for a count of at least sixteen.

6.11   "If you practice this control
for six months, you will be a master;
after a year you will see brahman;
therefore you must work at it, ceaselessly.

6.12   "Inhaling the air is *puraka;*
holding it in as though in a filled pot
is what is called *kumbhaka;*
exhaling it is named *rechaka.*

"The control causes sweating:
that is its least interesting effect;
executed better, it causes trembling;
those who perform it best
gain the power of levitation:
the better they are, the higher they rise.

6.15   By practicing the control it is certain
that you are purifying your mind completely;
then your aura becomes visible
surrounding your body with light.

"The mind and the breath unite
and settle within the atman;
it is then, aided by the power provided by control,
that the adept's body is able to rise of itself.

6.18   "Through the knowledge acquired in this way
one gains deliverance

from the chain of rebirths;
one can then abandon
puraka and rechaka,
and restrict oneself to kumbhaka alone;
all sins will be wiped out
and one will possess the high knowledge.

6.19   "By means of pranayama
the mind becomes clear and subtle,
gray hair returns to its former color,
there is nothing one may not achieve!
This is why one must practice
control further, and always.

6.20   "If you practice control,
taking the air in deeply,
at dawn and at dusk,[26]
or before daybreak appears,
or at noon if you prefer,
hold your breath at the tip of your nose,
in your navel or your toes:
this will make you live a hundred years!

"For the breath is well tamed
if it is held at the tip of the nose;
if you hold it in your navel,
sickness will have no hold on you;
and if it is kept in the toes,
your body will become shining bright!

6.25   "Drink the air by inhaling it
through the mouth and using your tongue:
you will never be thirsty or hungry
and you will never know fatigue.

"If you keep the breath
at the root of your tongue,
you will be able to drink ambrosia
and will know true happiness.

"By drawing it in through the ida
and holding it between the eyebrows,
you will drink nectar and keep
your body in good health forever.

"By using the two nadis[27]
and guiding the air down to the navel,
you will be preserved from all sickness.

"And if, for a whole month,
you drink nectar drop by drop,
inhaling the air three times a day
and retaining it in accordance with the rules
in a chosen part of your body,
any sickness deriving from wind or bile
will never be able to affect you.

6.31   "Diseases of the eyes
are cured by breath held in the forehead[28]
just as diseases of the ears are cured
by breath held in the ears,
and headaches by breath
held at the base of the head.

6.32   "Thus seated in the position
known as the auspicious sign,
with his mind well controlled,
making apana rise gently within
and repeating the pranava,
the adept should use his hands
to cut himself off from the outside world;
his thumbs will close his ears,
his index fingers his eyes
and two other fingers his nostrils:
in this way he will hold the apana
right inside his head
until he knows joy,
for the breath will then have reached
the door of the brahmarandra.

6.36   "At this moment the Sound
            will suddenly manifest itself,
            as though a conch were being blown;
            then it will be like a roll of thunder,
            and when the breath finally reaches
            the very top of the head,
            you will hear the reverberation
            of a mountain waterfall,
            and your atman, taking pleasure in this sound,
            will in truth show himself to you. [. . .]²⁹

7.1   "Now listen
            to what is called withdrawal of the senses;
            it consists in forcing the senses,
            by violent means, to withdraw back into themselves,
            whereas their true nature
            is to disperse themselves outside us.

            "Moreover, the true withdrawal
            is to see brahman in all things,
            as the rishis taught.
            Whatever you do, whether good, whether bad,
            do it until the day of your death
            while perceiving brahman in it:
            that is withdrawal of the senses!

7.5   "Performing the ceremonial
            of solemn or domestic rites
            in accordance with the rules of the *Veda*
            while perceiving brahman in them:
            that is withdrawal of the senses!

            "You can also guide
            your breath from place to place within your body
            from your teeth to your throat,
            or from your throat to your chest,
            from your chest to your navel,
            and from the navel down to the muladhara
            where the kundalini lies;

down to your buttocks and your thighs,
down to your knees, your calves,
and right down to your toes:
that also is withdrawal!

7.10   "If you do these things
yours sins will vanish away,
your sicknesses will disappear,
as those who know teach [. . .]³⁰

8.1   "And now comes dharana
of which we know several kinds,
relating to the five elements
together with their homologues in the body:

"In the space within the body
external space should be held
and in the same way the air of outside
should be held in the prana,³¹
and fire in the fire-in-the-abdomen:
one should also hold the waters
in the liquids of one's body,
and earth in the earthly parts.³²
that is dharana, oh Samkriti!

8.3   "Pronounce the mantra
ya, ra, va, la, in the correct order:
this sort of dharana
will free you from sin.

"From the feet up to the knees
the body belongs to earth;
from knees to anus, it is water;
from there up to the heart it is fire,
and air up to the middle of the forehead;
the head belongs to space.³³

8.5   In earth one sees Brahma,
Vishnu in the aqueous part;

Maheshana[34] inhabits fire,
Ishvara the air
and Shiva that part of your body
governed by the element space!

8.7   "You may also, if you prefer,
         meditate solely on Shiva,
         in order to free yourself from all ill;
         you will see him in your atman,
         full of wisdom and joy,
         residing in purusha
         sole principle of this world.

8.9   "And with all your mind
         fixed on the non-manifested,
         the without-form, the indefinable,
         you will see it, the sole principle,
         in the form of the pranava
         which is no other than your atman:
         it is then, with your senses withdrawn,
         that you will become one with your atman!

9.1   "You will then pass on
         to deep meditation,
         by means of which are destroyed for ever
         the bonds of transmigration.

         "In all humility
         one meditates on the Lord,
         the brahman-truth-reality,
         the brahman-pure-transcendence!

         "In this way the true yogi,
         freed from the laws of existence,
         chaste forever and seeing all things,
         meditates upon Ishvara,
         realizing: 'I am He!'

9.3   "And you may also meditate
         on Ishana, the truth,

the non-dual knowledge,
pure, eternal, and without past
as well as without present or future;
subtle, inconceivable, unperceivable,
without smell or savor, unmeasurable;
the One that is no other than the soul,
being-consciousness-joy;
realizing: 'I am that brahman!'
you will achieve liberation!

10.1   "When there appears within you
the true knowledge of the unity
of your atman with the cosmic atman,
that is called samadhi,
for the atman is in truth
identical with brahman, the omnipresent,
the perpetual, the One without second.

"In this way you can realize
that its forms are illusory:
there is no duality,
no world of phenomena,
or any transmigration either!
Just as the space in the pot
is not differentiated from the space around you;
just so, there is but one atman
and only the ignorant call it
'living soul' or 'Ishvara.'

10.5   "You must say to yourself in truth:
I am not body, or vital breath,
or sense, or thought, or anything else;
for I am the unique observer,
I am Shiva! I am Shiva!

"Yes, I am Brahman;
I am a stranger to this world,
there is no one with me![35]
Just as the spume and the waves

are born of the ocean then melt back into it,
so the world is born of me and melts back into me!

10.7 "He who knows this
achieves immortality at a stroke
by becoming purusha.
And universal consciousness,
luminous and omnipresent,
radiates in his heart:
in this way he attains brahman.

10.9 "If he no longer sees anything but 'That,'
remaining forever in samadhi,
he is forever brahman
and perceives his soul in it;
the world then melts away:
joy alone remains!"

Dattatreya spoke no more,
and Samkriti, well satisfied,
took refuge in his soul
and felt anxiety no more.

Such is the *Upanishad*.

Notes

Introduction

1. Vishnu is one of the major gods forming the Hindu trinity. He is the guardian of the world and undergoes incarnation whenever it is necessary to save the world (doctrine of Vishnu's avatars).

The *Rig Veda* is one of the great divisions of the *Veda*. Translations by F. Max Müller and H. Oldenberg of some hymns from the *Rig Veda* appear in *Sacred Books of the East* (Oxford, 1897; reprinted 1965), vols. 32 and 46.

2. On Mohenjo-Daro, see Sir Mortimer Wheeler, *Civilization of the Indus Valley* (London: Thames and Hudson, 1966).

3. Hinduism's doctrine of the four ages of the world is very much the same as Hesiod's, and so for simplicity's sake the Greek names have been used here.

4. Sanskrit is an Indo-European language (and therefore closely related to Latin, Greek, ancient Slav, Germanic, Armenian, Hittite, Persian, the Celtic languages, etc.) that was spoken until about the seventh century B.C. and has survived up to our own days as the learned language used by the brahmins. See T. Burrow, *The Sanskrit Language* (London: Faber and Faber, 1955.

5. Pandits: the *literati*, brahmins specializing in the Sanskrit tradition. Hence English "pundit."

6. *Yoga-Sutras:* Mnemotechnical aphorisms concerning yoga. On this subject, consult H. Woods, *The Yoga Sutras Translated* (Cambridge: Harvard University Press, 1913).

7. Almost all the *Puranas* have been translated into English, e.g., J. M. Sanyal, *The Bhagavata Purana*, 5 vols. (Calcutta, 1950). The best of the English translations of the *Bhagavad-Gita* is that by F. Edgerton (Cambridge: Harvard University Press, 1944). A few *Tantras* have been translated into English by Arthur Avalon (Sir John Woodroffe). See, e.g., *The Great Liberation* (Madras, 1913; reprinted 1952). For the *Upanishads,* see R. E. Hume, *The Thirteen Principal Upanishads* (Oxford University Press, 1934).

8. The rope trick consisted in the yogi's throwing a rope up into the air so that it appeared to remain upright and rigid of its own accord. The yogi then climbed the rope and remained suspended in mid-air at the top of it.

Chapter 1. The Cosmic Order

1. Here the universal craftsman is compared to a smith, a sort of Vulcan.
2. Hymn from the *Rig Veda,* 10.80, stanza 3, dedicated to Vishvakarman.

3. *Rig Veda,* 10.81.4.

4. *Maha-Narayana Upanishad,* 1.3–5.

5. *Mundaka Upanishad,* 1.6. Complete translation in R. E. Hume (see above, Introduction, n. 7).

6. Hymn from the *Rig Veda,* 10.90, stanzas 1, 2, 13. Saying that Purusha has "a thousand heads," etc., is to emphasize his superhuman character.

7. Ramanuja: philosopher, theologian, and preacher (died 1137) who raised the metaphysics of devotion to intellectual respectability. See S. N. Das Gupta, *A History of Indian Philosophy,* 5 vols. (Cambridge University Press, 1951).

8. *Atharva Veda,* 10.7.

9. The word *ahimsa* was used by Gandhi to denote nonviolent revolutionary action (boycott, strike, fast). On this subject, see *Hindu Dharma* (Ahmedabad, 1950), a selection from Gandhi's religious writings.

10. Further information on these various deities may be found in A. A. Macdonell, *Vedic Mythology* (Strasbourg, 1897).

11. See A. Getty, *Ganesha, the Elephant-Faced God* (Oxford University Press, 1934).

12. The complete Indian flood legend can be found in J. Muir, *Original Sanskrit Texts,* vol. 1 (London, 1871; reprinted 1967).

13. Kali-Yuga is the last—and most debased—of the four cosmic ages equivalent to the Iron Age in Hesiod's *Theogony.*

14. Parvati is called "the mountain goddess" because, like Shiva, she loves the rocky, ice-covered peaks so propitious to solitary meditation.

Chapter 2.   Man as Analogue

1. On these modern Hindu masters, see D. S. Sharma, *The Renaissance of Hinduism* (Benares, 1944).

2. The word "caste" is not Indian but of Portuguese origin. The best book in question is Louis Dumont, *Homo Hierarchicus: The Caste System and Its Implications* (University of Chicago Press, 1970).

3. The best account of the system of *gunas* occurs in the *Samkhya-Karikas* by Ishvara Krishna, written at the very beginning of the Christian era. There is a well-annotated English translation by D. H. Sharma, *The Samkhya-Karikas* (Poona, 1933).

4. George Dumézil's entire work over the past half-century has been devoted to researching the socioreligious evidence on the threefold ideology of the Indo-Europeans contained in ancient texts, rituals, myths, etc. See, e.g., *The Destiny of the Warrior* and *The Destiny of a King,* both translated by Alf Hiltebeitel (University of Chicago Press, 1970, 1973).

5. Aryan (from the Sanskrit *arya,* "noble") is another word for Indo-European. However, it refers more precisely to those Indo-European tribes which came into India about 1800 B.C. and finally settled in Iran and Punjab. They were the bearers of what was to become the Brahmanic civilization.

6. *Upanayana:* the ceremony that marks the entry of the young Hindu

(between the ages of eight and twelve) into the adult community. Until that age he has been raised by the women of the house in their quarters, which he now leaves in order to begin his studies and prepare himself for his "normal" (i.e., in accordance with dharma) life as head of a household.

7. It was the pariahs that Gandhi attempted to rehabilitate by giving them the name of harijans (people of God). As we know, modern India legally suppressed untouchability in 1949, but popular attitudes have scarcely been affected.

8. Heart of the earth: India itself, considered as the Holy Land, and more particularly the Kurukshetra, the narrow plateau to the south of Delhi between the Ganges and Indus valleys.

9. The marriage ritual includes one element that is particularly significant in this respect: the young couple are separated by a veil that is lifted only at a given point in the ceremony. And this is the instant, in theory at least, at which bride and groom see one another for the first time.

10. We read in the *Manava Dharma-Shastra,* for example: "The husband should make love with his wife at the prescribed times and remain faithfully attached to her; except during her monthly periods he should take his pleasure with her, drawn to her by the desire she inspires in him" (3.45).

11. Krishna's love affairs with the *gopis* (cow girls, milkmaids) and Radha provide the entire subject matter of the *Gita-Govinda,* translated into English by George Keyt as *The Song of Love* (Thompson, Conn.: Inter-Culture Associates, 1969).

12. "Wife" in Sanskrit is *bharya,* "she who must be supported, sustained, kept."

13. *Manava Dharma-Shastra,* 9.69 ff. It must be understood here that, in the eyes of Hindu tradition, marriage is primarily a contract, and the betrothal is therefore the decisive moment. Nowadays, in order to avoid the situation quoted here, the betrothal ritual is celebrated immediately before the marriage proper.

14. A man's profession often coincides with his jati. The smith caste, for example, is extremely likely to constitute a sort of trade guild. But this is not an absolute rule; Gandhi belonged to the perfume-maker's caste (that is the meaning of the word *gandhi*), but he was in fact a lawyer.

Chapter 3. Sarvam Duhkham

1. This was particularly true of Schopenhauer, who said in his *Parerga* that he had found confirmation in the *Upanishads* of his own philosophic pessimism.

2. *Maya* means, primarily, "measure," evoking the work of Vishvakarman, great architect of the universe, who fixed the measurements of the world. But in the *Veda* it has already taken on the meaning of phenomenal fantasmagoria. In the doctrine of Shankara (seventh century after Christ), maya is the cosmic illusion.

3. Every Hindu selects from the Hindu pantheon the divinity that best

corresponds with his temperament and then devotes an almost exclusive cult to that god; this is the *ishta-devata,* a man's "chosen god." Usually this divinity is also the family god, and the cult is passed on from father to son.

4. Prajapati, "Lord of creatures," is another name for Vishvakarman. Time is therefore higher than the creating God.

5. Lines from hymns 19, 53, and 54 of the *Atharva-Veda.* See also M. Bloomfield, *Hymns from the Atharva Veda* (Sacred Books of the East, vol. 42, Oxford University Press, 1897; reprinted 1965).

6. Ashoka (273–232 B.C.) was the first emperor of India–in other words, the first sovereign capable of creating political unity within the subcontinent to his own advantage.

7. *Maha Narayana Upanishad,* 10.10.1.

8. *Yogatattva Upanishad,* 1.10, 1.11.

9. *Bhagavad-Gita,* 2.20.

10. Ibid., 2.22.

11. *Yogatattva Upanishad,* 1.31 ff.

12. *Bhagavad-Gita,* 8.18, 8.19.

13. *Dhyanabindu Upanishad,* 1.5–1.7.

14. *Manava Dharma-Shastra,* 11.

15. Ibid., 12.56, 12.65.

16. Ibid., 12.16, 12.17.

Chapter 4.   Knowledge

1. This form of metaphysical pessimism is not a characteristic exclusive to Hinduism; it is a constant in everything Indian, as a look at Buddhism shows. We know, for instance, that Buddha's first sermon had as its theme the necessity–to which we are all subject–of undergoing the sorrows of existence: disease, age, death.

2. The "golden embryo" (*hiranya-garbha*) is at the same time an egg (the egg of Brahma). Breaking its shell in two, the Demiurge makes one into the earth, the other into the vault of heaven.

3. The primordial sacrifice is recounted in the *Rig Veda,* hymn 10.90. See A. A. Macdonell (above, chap. 1, n. 10).

4. "Magic": *maya,* which here is not, let me repeat, the "cosmic illusion," but the totality of the very real phenomena from which existence is woven.

5. *Yogatattva Upanishad,* 1.5, 1.6.

6. *Amritabindu Upanishad,* 1.18–1.20.

7. We read in book 7 of the *Chandogya Upanishad:* "Just as the spokes of a chariot wheel are all embodied in the hub of it, so living beings are all held in place by brahman, which is life."

8. *Amritabindu Upanished,* 1.17.

9. The primary meaning of *guru* is "heavy," "massive," the idea being that the master is weighty with a wealth of knowledge.

10. The prayer is female, though not *to* a female. Here it is in translation:

"May we receive the revelation of the Inciter's desirable light! May he spur our thoughts!" *Rig Veda*, 3.62.10.

11. Hindu tradition locates this third eye (symbolically, of course) either between the two "natural" eyes or "in the heart." The latter location is a reminder that the knower is the atman, which radiates its light "from within the heart."

12. Hindu tradition does not shrink from all the logical consequences of this situation. For example, since initiation is a birth, at the moment of upanayana the guru is proclaimed to be "pregnant" with his disciple.

13. See *The Gospel of Shri Ramakrishna,* translated by swami Nikhilan-anda (Madras, 1947).

14. Tantrism (from *tantra,* book) is the name given to that branch of Hinduism which gives predominance to the action of shakti, or cosmic energy, both in man and in the universe (see chap. 10).

Chapter 5.   *The Migratory Bird*

1. *Savitri,* it will be remembered, denotes the dawn prayer (*Rig Veda,* 3.62.10) communicated by master to pupil at the moment of the first (child-hood) initiation.

2. The Vedanta is one of the ten great systems of Hindu thought (dar-shanas) and the one that gives primacy among the instruments of liberation to the acquisition of knowledge.

3. *Kshurika Upanishad,* 1.22.

4. *Dhyanabindu Upanishad,* 1.62.

5. *Bhagavad-Gita,* 18.47. In this stanza Krishna is warning Arjuna against the error he would be committing if he tried to act not as the warrior he is but like a brahmin (for example) on the pretext that brahmins are metaphysically superior to warrior-nobles.

6. *Bhagavad-Gita,* 3.5.

7. *Manava Dharma-Shastra,* 12.3 The expression "bear fruit" is constantly employed in the traditional texts to depict the consequences of an act.

8. *Atharva Veda,* 9.2.19 ff.

9. *Bhagavad-Gita,* 3.12.

10. *Agnihotra:* offering of milk poured into the household fire during an extremely elaborate ritual ceremony.

11. *Yogatattva Upanishad,* 1.6.

12. *Kshurika Upanishad,* 1.25.

13. *Bhagavad-Gita,* 4.20.

14. Ibid., 3.40–3.42.

Chapter 6.   *From Yogas to Yoga*

1. The Sanskrit word for "yoke" is *yuga,* which is also the word used to denote each of the four periods or ages of the cosmic cycle.

2. *Mantra:* a ritual formula used in ceremonial liturgy or in operations of mental alchemy that will be referred to in later chapters.

3. A general account of the darshanas and Hindu philosophy as a whole will be found in M. Hiriyanna, *The Essentials of Indian Philosophy* (London, 1949).

4. *Bhagavad-Gita,* 18.56.

5. Ibid., 18.55.

6. *Katha-Upanishad,* 3.3. The best English translation of this text is that by R. E. Hume (see above, Introduction, n. 7).

7. *Bhagavad-Gita,* 3.41. Desire affects everything in the sphere of action, from the stimulus to action provided by the buddhi to its execution by the motor organs (indriya).

8. The doctrine of Vishnu's *avataras* or "descents."

9. *Bhagavad-Gita,* 3.39 (quoted in chapter 5).

10. *Yoga-Sutras,* 1.2.

11. *Atharva Veda,* 10.2.

Chapter 7. Taming the Body

1. As we shall see later, the fact of being accepted as disciple by a guru presupposes the fulfillment of conditions similar to those stipulated by Western religious orders; the body, in particular, must be whole and functioning normally in all its parts.

2. *Jivan-mukta:* "liberated-alive," meaning the man who has achieved liberation within the world of existence.

3. Sanskrit *ashrama:* "effort, place in which one strives for spiritual realization." Ashram is the modern form of the ancient word.

4. As in the case of Shri Aurobindo's ashram at Pondicherry, for example.

5. *Dvija:* "twice-born"—a high-caste Hindu who has undergone as a child the initiation of upanayana, which is held to be a "second birth."

6. So many works describe the life of the sadhus in such poetic language that the Western reader is filled with envy at the thought of such a delightful bucolic existence. But that reader can be in for a terrible shock if he eventually visits India for himself and chances to meet some of these appalling emaciated beings by the roadside or even to find them lying dead of hunger on the sunscorched ground.

7. See above, Introduction, n. 5.

8. See above, chap. 5, n. 10.

9. *Shiva-Samhita,* 3.13.

10. Ibid., 3.15.

11. Ibid., 3.11.

12. Ganesha has an elephant's head and is said to watch over intellectual labors.

13. The word *zen* is directly derived, by a simple phonetic shift, from the Chinese *tchan,* itself derived from Sanskrit *dhyana.*

14. *Shiva-Samhita*, 5.239 ff. "On its secret"; i.e., on the esoteric meaning of the mantra (see chap. 10).

15. *Yoga-Sutras*, 246.

16. For example, the Maharishi Mahesh Yogi (see Conclusion).

17. Théodore Brosse, *Etudes instrumentales des techniques du yoga* (Paris: Maisonneuve, 1963; available only in French).

Chapter 8.   Dissolving the Mind

1. "Impregnations" that have soaked deeply into our minds and determine our behavior in the conditions of everyday life.

2. Patanjali: the mythical author of the *Yoga-Sutras*. See Mircea Eliade, *Patanjali and Yoga* (New York: Funk and Wagnall, 1969).

3. The *Yoga Darshana Upanishad*, given in full at the end of this book, teaches a specific posture in which the yogi closes his eyes, ears, and nostrils with his hand (6.32).

4. *Mandala*: literally "circle," but the word denotes any symbolic diagram that can be used as a support for meditation. See G. Tucci, *Theory and Practice of the Mandala* (London: Rider, 1969).

5. *Dhyanabindu Upanishad*, 1.19.

6. Ibid., 1.23.

7. *Nadabindu Upanishad*, 1.40. *Pranava* is a Sanskrit word denoting the syllable *om*.

8. *Kshurika Upanishad*, 1.22.

Chapter 9.   Seeing God Face to Face

1. "Yoga is the suppression of mental activity" (*Yoga-Sutras*, 1.2). See above, Introduction.

2. *Yoga Darshana Upanishad*, 9.3. The full text of this *Upanishad* is given at the end of the book.

3. *Shiva-Samhita*, 3.63, 3.64.

4. *Yogatattva-Upanished*, 1.77, 1.78.

5. Ibid., 1.106.

6. Ibid., 1.108.

7. *Yogakundalini Upanishad*, 1.76–1.78.

8. See, for example, *Bhagavad-Gita*, 18.54.

9. A yogi's tomb is also termed a samadhi. The samadhi of Gandhi in Delhi, that of Aurobindo at Pondicherry, etc., are still venerated today.

10. Kundalini: name of the mysterious power present in all beings (see following chapters).

Chapter 10.   The Divine Couple

1. It will be remembered that one of the names for the cosmic energy invoked at the moment of initiation is *savitri*, the "Incitress."

2. See above, chap. 2, n. 5.

3. Particularly in the form given to maya by Shankara (eighth century after Christ).

Chapter 11.   The Subtle Body

1. "Informed": in the sense of "structured from within."

2. "Gods of the fields": the lower-ranking gods who preside over rural activities.

3. The prophets (*rishis*) are the holy men who revealed the *Veda* teachings, and the monks (*munis*) are the various kinds of sadhus.

4. *Shiva-Samhita,* 2.1–2.5.

5. *Dhyababindu-Upanishad,* 1.34.

6. *Yogatattva-Upanishad,* 1.85 ff.

Chapter 12.   The Power of the Serpent

1. *Yogakundalini Upanishad,* 1.82.

2. *Amritanada Upanishad,* 1.19.

3. Whenever a triangle figures in any of the chakras, it is always pointing downward, thus making it clear that feminine symbolism is predominant in the anatomy of the subtle body.

4. The syllable *om* is the mantra specific to the sixth chakra. Here the specific mantra is in fact *yam,* but all sounds are ultimately derived from the vibration of the eternal word, *om.*

5. Shiva-Samhita, 1.196.

6. Kailasa: a mythical mountain. Its "earthly" analogue is a Himalayan peak, the source of the Ganges.

Conclusion

1. See Sir Mortimer Wheeler, *The Indus Civilization* (Cambridge University Press, 1953).

2. See Mircea Eliade (above, chap. 8, n. 2).

3. Shri Aurobindo's works are published by his ashram in Pondicherry.

4. On Ramana Maharshi, see P. Brunton, *A Search in Secret India* (London, 1938).

The Yoga Darshana Upanishad

1. Usually the "great yogi" is Shiva; and it will be found that the *Upanishad* does advocate (10.5) identification with Shiva, not with Vishnu.

2. In the Bhagavad-Gita it is likewise Vishnu, in the guise of Krishna, who instructs Arjuna in yoga.

3. This identification of reality with what is perceived by the senses is certainly surprising. Later, however, the *Upanishad* says that the world of phenomena is nothing but illusion (10.3).

4. A veiled attack on the nihilist (*nastika*) Buddhists. The position yoga

takes is that the world is "existence" and not "nothingness" (or "vacuity," as the Buddhists say).

5. The theme of the master as "tempter," putting his disciple's submission to the test.

6. *Japa*—the constant repetition of a ritual formula. The best is that in which the prayer is not even murmured but simply "thought."

7. *Sukha*. As we know, the best position, according to the *Yoga-Sutras,* is the one that any particular practitioner finds "stable and relaxed" (*sthira-sukha*).

8. The muladhara chakra does in fact contain a downward-pointing triangle enclosed in a square.

9. "Knot-of-the-navel": probably the manipura chakra.

10. "Seventy-two thousand": a symbolic figure signifying a vast and indefinite number.

11. Brahma-nadi: the channel of brahman (because it leads up to the *brahmarandra,* the "brahman orifice" located at the very top of the skull.

12. *Ahamkara*—the inner force that causes us to say "I" (*aham*).

13. There are only five vital breaths in the more usual tradition.

14. "Hole-of-brahman": the orifice of brahman (the fontanel).

15. "Northern path": the path of the sun in winter.

16. The meeting point of the two "rivers" here would seem to be the top of the head.

17. Kedara: a Hymalayan peak; also the name of a spring that rises there.

18. The confluence of the Ganges and the Yamuna (the site of present-day Allahabad) is one of India's principal places of pilgrimage.

19. Kamalalaya: an unidentified tirtha.

20. The word *tirtha* applies primarily to the sacred Indian fords, but it can be used more generally to mean any stretch of water where ablutions can be made.

21. Practitioners of yoga are often referred to as *atma-yajins,* "those who take their own selves as god."

22. "Great mystery": the knowledge of brahman.

23. *Bilva:* wild apple tree sacred to Shiva.

24. "Eternal Sound": brahman manifesting itself as sound, in the form of the syllable *om.*

25. Pranava: the name of the syllable *om.*

26. Dawn and dusk are the two times of day when Hindu religious ceremonies are obligatory.

27. "The two nadis": the ida and the pingala.

28. That is, by channeling the prana to the ajna-chakra between the eyebrows.

29. The final stanzas of this *khanda* are too corrupt for adequate translation.

30. Again there are a number of very corrupt stanzas.

31. The idea here is that the prana remains permanently in man's body throughout his life; the air inhaled simply sets it in motion.

32."Earthly parts": those governed by the element earth.

33. *Akasha,* which can also be translated as "ether."

34. Maheshana: one of the names of Shiva.

35. "There is no one with me": *kaivalya,* the state of absolute solitude that the *Yoga-Sutras* say is the goal of those who practice yoga.

Glossary

ahimsa (f.). Abstinence from causing any kind of injury to a living being.

ajna (f.), *ajna-chakra* (m.). Sixth center of the subtle body, located just above the eyebrows.

anahata (m.). Fourth center of the subtle body, located at heart level.

asana (m.). Posture; position of the body used for meditation.

ashrama (m.). Effort; the word from which modern "ashram" is derived—a collection of disciples around their spiritual master (*guru*).

atman (m.). Soul, eternal principle; identical with the Absolute (*brahman*) present at the heart of every living being. Sometimes translated as "self."

avatara (m.). Descent, avatar; an incarnation of Vishnu as a living being given the task of saving *dharma* when a demon endangers it. Vishnu's two most important *avatara* are Rama and Krishna.

bhakti-yoga (m.). Method of achieving salvation (*yoga*) through devotion (*bhakti*). This is the yoga preached by Krishna in the *Bhagavad-Gita*.

brahman (m.). The Absolute, the sole principle of all things, the transcendent essence of all the forms of existence. Identical with *atman*.

buddhi (f.). Intelligence, highest element of the human composite.

Its principal function is to reflect down onto the mind (*manas*) the light emanating from the atman.

chakra (m.). Wheel, circle. Name given to the seven centers of the subtle body, which are also called *padma* (lotuses).

chitta (neut.). Mental activity, which it is yoga's aim to arrest.

darshana (neut.). Point of view, way of looking; generic name given to the great schools of Hindu thought (yoga, Vedanta, etc.).

dharana (f). Perfect concentration; the sixth stage of yoga, the object of which is the dissolution of the mind (*manas*).

dharma (m.). Denotes the order governing the cosmos in all its manifestations (cosmic, social, religious, etc.); also classical Hinduism's traditional laws as a totality.

dhyana (neut.). Meditation; seventh stage of yoga, the object of which is to enable the practitioner to "see" his atman (and thus achieve *samadhi*, the final stage before liberation).

dvija (m.). Twice-born; denotes those Hindus entitled to *upanayana*, i.e., high-caste Hindus as opposed to *shudras* and *pariahs*.

ekagrata (f.). Concentration of the attention on a single point; state achieved by means of breath control and sense withdrawal in preparation for the attainment of *dharana*.

guna (m.). Quality, attribute; used to denote the world's three modes of existence, which are hierarchized in accordance with their distance from the Absolute: *tamas* (darkness), *rajas* (passion, activity), *sattva* (harmony with being).

guru (m.). Weighty, important; name given by a disciple or disciples to a *sadhu* when he agrees to become their teacher.

hamsa (m.). Migratory bird; symbol of the soul condemned to transmigrate from body to body until the end of the cosmic cycle.

hatha-yoga (m.). Method of attaining salvation (*yoga*) employing physical energy (*hatha*). *Hatha-yoga* emphasizes the mastering of difficult postures.

ida (f.). One of the three principal *nadis*. It is yellow and linked with the Ganges and the moon.

indriya (neut.). Of or like Indra, the king of creation; in humans denotes the motor functions and the organs and faculties of sense.

japa (m.). Repetition; devotional exercise consisting in the indefinite repetition of a *mantra* or the name of a diety; in *bhakti-yoga,* a technique for the dissolution of thought.

jati (f.). Birth, caste (subdivision of *varna*).

jiva (m.). Living; abbreviation for *jiva-atman* (living soul), which denotes the soul when embodied.

jivan-mukta (m.). Liberated-alive; a yogi who has reached the final stage of yoga.

jnana-yoga (m.). Method of achieving salvation (*yoga*) principally by the pursuit of intellectual knowledge (*jnana*).

kaivalya (neut.). Isolation; the state of the individual when his entire being has been reabsorbed into *atman brahman,* the sole principle of all things.

kali-yuga (m.). Fourth and last period of cosmic development, the iron age, which immediately precedes the dissolution of the universe.

kama (m.). Love, desire; prime motor of existence; yoga sets out to eliminate it so that the *atman* can return to essence.

karman (neut.). Act, work, action; according to yoga, every action performed by the individual produces an effect and leaves behind a psychic residue (also called *karman*) which imprisons the soul in the world of existence.

karma-yoga (m.). Method of achieving salvation (*yoga*) through disinterested action (*karman*); Krishna preaches a combination of *karma-yoga* and *bhakti-yoga* in the *Bhagavad-Gita.*

kshatriya (m.). Hindu belonging to a caste related to the "second function" (warriors, nobles, etc.).

kundalini (f.). coiled; the female serpent coiled up in the cave at the base of the subtle body (symbol of the cosmic power or *shakti* present in every living being).

linga (neut.). Erect phallus; the symbol of Shiva's power over nature and living beings. It is worshiped (in the shape of an erect stone) in Shivaite temples or shrines.

manas (m.). Mind, thought; mental organ (brain) and its function (thought). Yoga uses it to harness all the individual's vital energies, then attempts to dissolve it in order to reach a higher level, that of the *buddhi* or cosmic intelligence.

mandala (neut.). Disk, geometric figure; denotes the diagrams often used as aids to meditation.

manipura (neut.). Third center of the subtle body, located at navel level.

mantra (neut.). Tool of thought, ritual formula (secret and given during initiation) used as an aid to meditation.

maya (f.). Magic; cosmic power whose function is the unfurling of the infinitely varied forms of existence.

moksha (m.). Liberation; freeing of the captive soul from phenomenal existence. pp. 73, 174 ff. 110, 265.

mukti (f.). Synonymous with *moksha*.

muladhara (m.). First center of the subtle body located at anus level.

nadi (f.). River; symbolic term for channels through which the "vital breath" circulates in the subtle body.

niyama (m.). Spiritual discipline; second stage of yoga, aimed at leading the novice toward the practice of certain virtues.

om. Sacred syllable that is brahman itself as sound. It is made up of the three sounds *a, u, m,* which in accordance with the phonetic rules of Sanskrit merge into one: *o* prolonged into a reverberation notated as *m*.

padma (m.). Lotus; another term for the centers of the subtle body or *chakras*.

padma-asana (m.). Lotus position, one of the most famous postures used in meditation.

pingala (f.). One of the three principal *nadis* (red, and linked with the Yamuna river and the sun).

prakriti (f.). Matter, nature, as opposed to spirit (*purusha*), with which it forms a god/goddess couple.

prana (m.). Plenitude; name given to the "vital breath" and by extension to the air physically inhaled.

pranava (m.). Resonance, used to designate the syllable *om*.

pranayama (m.). Control of the breath; fourth stage of yoga, consisting in regulating one's breathing in order to slow it down, then in holding the breath inhaled for as long as possible.

pratyahara (m.). Withdrawal (of the senses); fifth stage of yoga, consisting in screening the mind against all external stimuli.

purusha (m.). Male; used to denote spirit as opposed to matter (*prakriti*), which is female.

raja-yoga (m.). Royal art; denotes yoga as such, as opposed to ancillary methods such as *bhakti-yoga,* etc.

rishi (m.). Prophet, seer; one of the mythical personages who received the original revelation of the Hindu scriptures.

rita (neut.). Ordered, fitted together; archaic term for *dharma*.

sach-chid-ananda (neut.). Being-consciousness-joy, a tria describing the true nature of *brahman*.

sadhu (m.). Saint; name given to those who have renounced the world in order to follow the path leading to the Absolute.

sahasrara (m.). Seventh and last center of the subtle body, symbolized by a thousand-spoked wheel or a thousand-petaled lotus.

samadhi (m.). Eighth and last stage of yoga, in which the *atman* achieves liberation, thus enabling the practitioner to attain the state of ontological isolation called *kaivalya*.

samsara (m). The flow to which all things are subjected; the universal law of the transmigration of the soul from body to body during any one entire cosmic cycle.

savitri (f.). Incitress; a name constituting the *mantra* given to the "twice-born" at the moment of *upanayana*. The high-caste Hindu should repeat it at least three times a day.

shakti (f.). Power; divine energy, representation of the true nature of all the major gods; in men, *shakti* takes the form of the *kundalini*.

shudra (m.). Servant; name given to Hindus who, though not outcastes, are nevertheless excluded from *upanayana* and therefore are not entitled to the title *dvija*.

siddhi (f.). Accomplishment, achievement; used to denote the miraculous powers acquired through the practice of yoga.

sushumna (f.). The most important of the three principal *nadis* (linked with the river Sarasvati).

svadhishthana (m.). Second center of the subtle body, at the level of the genitals.

tad (neut.). "That"; metaphysical term for the Absolute (*atman/ brahman*).

tirtha (neut.). Sacred place; usually refers to the bank of a river where people gather for ritual bathing.

upanayana (neut.). Initiation ceremony undergone by all young high-caste Hindu males at about the age of seven.

vaishya (m.). People belonging to the "third function" (production, finance, crafts) who are permitted initiation and thus entitled to the title *dvija*.

varna (m.). Color; used to denote the three broad functions among which the numerous castes (*jatis*) are divided.

vasana (f.). Impregnation; the residual trace left by any act (or thought); cause of the metaphysical ignorance that produces alienation.

vibhuti (f.). Another word for *siddhis* (miraculous powers).

vishuddha (m.). Fifth center of the subtle body, located at throat level.

yama (m.). Restraint; first stage of yoga, during which the novice strives to put behind him the disturbing influence of worldly things.

yantra (neut.). A restraining instrument; a geometric figure used as an aid to meditation (synonymous with *mandala*).

Suggestions for Further Reading

The number of books about India, Hinduism, Yoga, and Tantrism is enormous. Since there can be no question of listing them all here, I have merely signposted a few paths that will lead the reader a little deeper into the subject, should he or she wish to follow them. And for anyone who wishes to go even farther, each of the works listed below will be found to contain a more specialized bibliography.

General Works

The following general books have a slight emphasis on cultural aspects of India:

Hurlimann, Martin. *India.* London: Thames and Hudson, 1967. (A collection of excellent photographs.)
Spate, O. H. C. *India and Pakistan: A General and Regional Geography.* With the collaboration of A. M. Learmonth and a chapter on Ceylon by B. H. Farmer. 3d ed. London: Methuen, 1967.

History of India

The two best histories of India in English are:

Allan, John; Haig, T. Wolseley; and Dodwell, H. H. *The Cambridge Shorter History of India.* Edited by H. H. Dodwell. Cambridge University Press, 1934. Reprinted, Mystic, Conn.: Lawrence Verry, 1969.
Smith, Vincent A. *The Oxford History of India.* 2d ed. Edited by Percival Spear. Oxford University Press, 1958.

Among other works are:

Davies, Cuthbert C. *An Historical Atlas of the Indian Peninsula.* Bombay: Indian Branch, Oxford University Press, 1949.
Panikkar, K. M. *A Survey of Indian History.* 4th ed. New York: Asia Publishing House, 1964.

Rawlinson, Hugh G. *India: A Short Cultural History*. New York: Praeger, 1952.

Indian Civilization

For a general view of Indian civilization in classical times there is one admirable and indispensable book:

Basham, Arthur L. *The Wonder That Was India: A Survey of the Culture of the Indian Sub-continent before the Coming of the Muslims*. Rev. ed. New York: Hawthorn Books, 1963.

Worth mentioning also are:

Lannoy, Richard. *The Speaking Tree: A Study of Indian Culture and Society*. London and New York: Oxford University Press, 1971.
Masson-Oursel, Paul; Willman Grabowska, Helena de; and Stern, Philippe. *Ancient India and Indian Civilization*. Translated by M. R. Dobie. New York: Barnes and Noble, 1967.

The caste problem has been dealt with in English by a number of authors, including:

Dumont, Louis. *Homo Hierarchicus: The Caste System and Its Implications*. University of Chicago Press, 1970.
Hutton, John H. *Caste in India: Its Nature, Function, and Origins*. 4th ed. London: Indian Branch, Oxford University Press, 1963.
Marriott, McKim, and Inden, Ronald. "Caste." In *Encyclopaedia Britannica*, 15th ed. 1974.
Zinkin, Taya, *Caste Today*. London and New York: Oxford University Press, 1962.

Hinduism

The most convenient book is:

Zaehner, Robert C. *Hinduism*. London and New York: Oxford University Press, 1962.

Among many others, I would select:

Daniélou, Alain. *Hindu Polytheism*. Princeton University Press, 1964.
Eliot, Charles N. E. *Hinduism and Buddhism: An Historical Sketch*. London: Routledge and Kegan Paul, 1964.

Renou, Louis. *Religions of Ancient India.* New York: Schocken, 1968.

Anthologies of Hindu scriptures in English translation include:

Muir, John, ed. and tr. *Original Sanskrit Texts on the Origin and History of the People of India, Their Religion and Institutions.* London, 1872–74.
Renou, Louis, ed. *Hinduism.* New York: George Braziller, 1961.

Tantrism

The most authoritative works are those of Sir John Woodroffe (pseudonym: Arthur Avalon), constantly reprinted in India by Ganesh and Company, Madras. Three such reprints are:

Shakti and Shakta: Essays and Addresses on the Shakta Tantrashastra. 6th ed. 1965.
The Serpent Power. 7th ed. 1964.
The World as Power. 3rd ed. 1966.

Other available books are:

Agehananda Bharati. *The Tantric Tradition.* London: Rider, 1965. Paperback ed., New York: Doubleday, 1970.
Rawson, Philip S. *The Art of Tantra.* Greenwich, Conn.: New York Graphic Society, 1973.
Tucci, Giuseppe. *The Theory and Practice of the Mandala, with Special Reference to the Modern Psychology of the Unconscious.* Translated by A. H. Brodrick. London: Rider, 1969.
Wayman, Alex. *The Buddhist Tantras: Light on Indo-Tibetan Esotericism.* New York: Weiser, 1973.

Yoga

If anything, there have been rather too many books published on the subject recently. Keeping exclusively to scholarly works (and being very selective among those), I would mention:

Das Gupta, S. N. *Yoga as Philosophy and Religion.* London: K. Paul, Trench, Trubner, 1924; New York: Dutton, 1924.
Eliade, Mircea. *Yoga: Immortality and Freedom.* Translated from the French by W. R. Trask. 2nd ed. Princeton University Press, 1969.
Evola, Giulio C. A. *Lo yoga della potenza.* Milan: Fratelli Boca, 1949.

(A French translation has been published in Paris by Fayard under
the title *Le yoga tantrique*.)

Basic Yoga Texts

All the basic texts have been translated into English; some, such as
the *Bhagavad Gita,* have appeared in several translations, of which only
the best are listed here.

The Bhagavad Gita. Translated by Franklin Edgerton. Harvard University Press, 1944.

The Bhagavad Gita. Translated by Robert C. Zaehner. Oxford University Press, 1969.

The Gheranda Samhita. Translated by Srisa Chandra Vasu. 1914.
Reprinted, New York: AMS Press, 1974.

The Hatha Yoga Pradipika. Translated by Pancham Sinh. 1915. Reprinted, New York: AMS Press, 1974.

Upanishads du yoga. Translated by Jean Varenne. Paris: Gallimard,
1974. (A French translation of eight of the *Upanishads*.)

The Yoga System of Patanjali. Translated by J. H. Woods. Harvard
Oriental Series, vol. 17. 1913. Reprinted, Mystic, Conn.: Lawrence
Verry, 1972.

The Yoga Upanishads. Translated by T. R. Shrinivasa Ayyangar. Edited by Pandit A. Mahadeva Sastri. Madras: Adyar Library, 1920.

Index